The Life I Was Dealt

Right When You Think You Can't Handle Anything Else

Annie B

iUniverse, Inc.
New York   Bloomington

iUniverse books may be ordered through booksellers or by contacting:

iUniverse
1663 Liberty Drive
Bloomington, IN 47403
www.iuniverse.com
1-800-Authors (1-800-288-4677)

ISBN: 978-1-4401-2506-5 (sc)
ISBN: 978-1-4401-2508-9 (dj)
ISBN: 978-1-4401-2507-2 (ebook)

Library of Congress Control Number: 2009923493

Printed in the United States of America

iUniverse rev. date: 02/20/2009

Who am I.

I am my Mothers child. I started my life and learned the lessons she chose to teach. In her day her Mother never thought to discuss men and relationships with her. My Mother followed her example.

We each live a life unique. Our stories are the history of a life. It is said that we should learn from history. Not all of the history of my life is for others to learn from, what I did wrong. I did nothing wrong, I just didn't have sufficient maturity and knowledge about people, men, to make a more educated discussion.

Mike was my first real relationship. The abuse he dealt out I took out of ignorance, this is what happens. David was the same treatment, not as often or as severe, but still what to me was becoming the norm. Facing abusive relationships and trying life experiences becomes educational process. Instead of accepting abuse as ok, just what life is all about; I choose to learn to live a better life.

I hope by reading my story I can educate other women that they can change their lives. This is also a catharsis for me. You don't get rid of pain by holding on to it. On the pages that follow read my words, learn from my lessons. Don't feel sorry for me, I don't. When you get introduced to William you will see that two wrongs can be followed by a right.

Walk a mile in my high heels. It hurts to walk in heels but women still love them. They are a part of who we are.

The writing of this book was very difficult emotionally. The incidences were born of life experiences. I would like to thank my friend and companion William for helping find some of the words inside of me, and on some other occasions giving me the words to write.

Foreward

The weather was balmy, the sun sparkling on the ocean as a scrumptious breakfast was served on the patio of our villa. Life was good. The atmosphere seemed serene as friends enjoyed the beginning of a new day.

This was not so for Annie. The conversation turned to sharing stories about incidents at Baltimore Trade Center then to the World Trade Center in New York.

Annie cried silently with tears on her cheeks. She excused herself from the table with no explanations as talk continued.

This story may be considered a catharsis of our author's soul. Writing and talking has always been a way to make personal burdens seem lighter. Her style was to internalize her feelings, be quiet about her challenges and "move on". She radiates a sense of loving life with a smile on her face, a quick laugh and a clever speedy "come backs" in conversation. All seemed just right with her world.

The author shares her story of multitude challenges. The reader can be more empathic of how circumstances have incredible influence. Annie's children are a primary concern, with her cell phone always on frequent calls back and forth. Her Mother, far from "motherly", Annie always treats her with respect.

Annie's objective is for readers to know there can be a new beginning many times over.

Annie's Friend

Emily

My Life

I have spent many years of my life trying to figure out who I am.

It has been hard for me to accept who I am and be happy with it.

Years ago I read the scripture, "A gentle and quiet spirit is precious in the eyes of the Lord"...

After I read that, I felt bad about myself... for I wasn't gentle or quiet...

So I was determined to be "gentle and quiet".... literally...

I didn't talk much and I became a wall flower....

Thankfully, I realized that verse wasn't talking about my personality but my "spirit"...

God doesn't fit in a box....He created me in his own image... why should *I* fit in a box.

I am eclectic in my music, personal style and hobbies...

I have my share of "critics"... people who have nothing better to do than to sit around and judge me and others different from themselves...

We don't fit in their expectations, or their idea of who we should be. After 38 years, I have learned to embrace who I am and not be ashamed. I want to be different than you or her... or her....

I am creative, I love all kinds of rock music, I do not want a tattoo, I like to be competitive, I am generous, I like to be outside, I am a hard worker....

I challenge you to discover who you are, and live it to the fullest....

"The Life I was Dealt"

Right When You Think You Can't Handle Anything Else

Settle

One of the most exciting and encouraging truths in life is that we can always become someone new. We never have to settle for who we are.

God gives those who can handle it challenges in Life; I don't understand why I keep coming to the front of the line.

Table of Contents

My Life iii

Growing up 1

My Daddy Family 3

Neighbors 8

Brother's and Sister's...11

Jr. High School 15

Sharing my Talents 19

Incredible Opportunity...21

Marriage to Mike while in High School 23

Move to California 25

360 - The Day it all Started 28

1st Try at Leaving...32

Is it safe to take a Shower? 38

The Unexpected...41

2nd Try at Leaving...43

The Worse Night Ever...45

After the Accident...47

Marriage to Mike is Over...50

Meeting David 53

Deshawn...56

Breast Cancer 64

Marriage to David 66

Kid's Talk..68

Abuse starts again...71

The next Move..74

Red, White – I'm Blue...76

Medical Trip 79

Home from Medical Trip 85

Last Tour Trip 87

Flight home after 911 94

Sept 19, 06 103

Oct 22, 06 107

WOW GOOD NEWS 116

David or Mike 118

Christmas '07' 120

Jan 08 122

Holding Hands 124

Talking with William 126

Hotel Shooting 128

Traveling with my Group 129

Talking with David 130

Surgery 133

Grape Stomp 135

Trip to Mexico 137

David 139

Closing 141

Modeling Events: 142

Some Additional Funny Stories 143

Love Letters and Text messages to Annie from William 147

Love Letters and Text Messages to WILLIAM from Annie B .162

Love Thoughts by others, ...184

How to Get in Touch With Me 188

Some of My Favorite Recepies

Chicken and Noodle Casserole 193

BBQ Bash Party Mix 194

White Chips and Blueberry Bread Pudding 195

First Class Coconut Cake...197

Texas Cow Chip Cookies 198

Volcano Cake 199

Pumpkin Cheesecake 200

Peppermint Stick Cheesecake 201

Chocolate Chip Cheesecake..202

Pralines and Cream Cheesecake...203

Onion Dip..204

Texas Two-Step Slaw 205

Sweet Potato Casserole..206

Western Baked Beans...207

Corn Casserole 208

Lickety Split Spoons 209

Pumpkin Pie..210

Yummy Chocolate Cake...211

Holiday Peppermint Bark..212

Taco Stew...213

Chilies Relleno's Casserole 214

Sweet – n – Sour Meatballs...215

Pork Chop Casserole 216

Chicken Taco's...217

Chicken Spaghetti...218
Chicken Tortilla Bake..219
Acorn Squash Casserole 220

Wow where does one begin...

Growing up

I would sit in my crib, or on mother's lap or in the middle of the floor, walling in amusement as eleven brothers and sisters came and went, yelling, screaming, laughing and teasing one another.

My Papa worked long hours and I think I must have been five or six before I understood who he was.

I was the baby in the family. I am number twelve out of twelve children; there are nine boys and three girls. When I lived at home I always knew that there was something very unusual about me, however I just could not distinguish yet what that something was.

You see my Mom is Irish, along with my Papa (that I'm familiar with) is Spanish. Therefore, when I say that I am different it is for the reason that each and every one of my brothers as well as my sisters are tanned, (Mexican American) and I am pale almost to the point of being an albino, with brilliant red curly hair.

While I was growing up, I constantly thought about all the family things that I did with this second family. They were pleasant and all, except I just did not comprehend why I was the only one from my family that I lived with, which had to go off and do things in the company of this other family.

Now looking back at it, it all makes more sense; each family is in fact my family, as well. One day I found out that they were my aunts, uncles and cousins from my natural father's side of the family.

It was not till I was in Jr. High School that I found out that my Mom had an affair, and I am the "Love Child" of that affair. That was when I was about twelve years old and I went to visit this other man and stayed with him and his wife. Eventually I learned that he was my Natural Daddy.

My Mom, at all times would make certain I attended these family gatherings from my Natural Father's side of the family. I just could never figure out how come none of my other brother's or sister's had to go.

But a child no matter how young doesn't complain about being spoiled by more than one family. This went on for years, then one day one of my brothers started going with me, I believe he was just feeling sorry for me.

Once I found out, I would go to my Dad's house and stay a week at a time, every once in a while. He lived about five hours away, in a little town called Beeville, down in the direction of San Antonio. Consequently I saw him more when he came into the town where I was living at the time. I was only able to go to his house over holidays and summer breaks.

My Daddy Family

Country folks and Country Gatherings. A sea of aunts, uncles, cousins, seniors and babies.

Men with Beer bellies and pregnant women. Sometimes you had to look at the faces to tell who was who. But they were Wonderful. Everyone brought something to share and everyone had their job. Conner did the barbequing and Robin; his wife critiqued his methods and results. Cousin Conner, the delegate cook, and actually a chef, was the Captain of the barbecue. If you could conceivably cook it over charcoal he did. Today there were two slabs of ribs, each over two feet long, and a brisket that was as large and weighed as much as some of the kids.

He added his spices and soaked it with sauce,

"Conner what are you doing?" Robin says.

His wife of forever, teenage boy and girlfriend, married for over thirty years.

Conner tells her:

"sprinkle the salt, pepper, and garlic don't coat it just sprinkle"

"Sugar"

"Everyone loved it last time; they'll love it again this time".

"I've been doing this forever, and no one has complained yet"

Robin says: "ok, master cook, then at least watch the sauce, the meat should have some taste it can call its own"

"Barbeque isn't about the meat, it's the flavor"

"I'm the flavor" says Conner

"And just make sure Sue has lots of Alka Seltzer and Maalox on hand"

The kids get hamburgers and hot dogs not much you can do to them.

Beth, the Queen of desserts, and Beverly keeping us all green and healthy with the salads. Ice chest filled to the brim with soda's and not a beer company without representation.

And the stories they would tell. The Barn while I was with this family, some of my male cousins and I would always find a moment to sneak away and we would always be found in the Barn. There was always some assumption about what we were up to, but no one would ever believe us this went on from about age six and carried on in to our teenage years, even when we told them we just wanted to get away from everything that was going on.

So even now when we have family gathers (and the Barn has now been torn down) everyone will talk about us going to the Barn. Whenever one of my cousins would get married they would ask their bride:

"Have they told you about their days in the Barn?"

I enjoyed going away to my Dad's house, he raised all kinds of farm animals, horses, sheep, pigs... you name it and he had it. As a result when I would go there I was able to help brush them all out, and take them for walks.

Occasionally we would go fishing, or go to his deer lease to get it prepared for the wintery weather months. Dad taught me to fish and like many things in my life I learned too well and exceeded expectations. One day when out fishing at the pond, I caught a twelve pound Catfish. I laid it next to Daddy's two – six ounce Croppies. Daddy grabbed his rod and threw it into the pond.

"Child I've had enough of your showing off"

"You can find someone else to go fishing with".

Years later it was a Golf Club that went flying when I beat him at that too. I will learn one day that men don't like to lose especially to a woman, let alone their daughter.

Daddy's daughter; became his buddy, and part time son. Part of it was the fact that I wasn't into all the dresses and lace. Daddy loves animals, but he truly loves to fish and hunt. Like the day he fell overboard while getting overly excited about the fish on the line, it was way too funny. He had on those fishing waders that had lots of pockets, they were filling up with water and he was going down. Once we finally got him back in the boat he realized he also had his phone in his pocket.

I asked him:

"Who did you think you were going to call Tuna Sr. to come get you out?"

He is now back in the boat

"Daddy did you at least catch anything?"

"After all you do have a lot of pockets there".

One of my favorite stories happened while at the Deer lease. When Daddy got to quick on the trigger. The day started early and we didn't see any deer most of the morning,

"Well little girl it looks like one of those days"

"The deer are in Oklahoma and we are hunting in Texas."

"Daddy give it a little more time!"

"We usually see something out there"

Daddy says:

"With our luck we'll only see Doe's and Ducks" "and we can't shoot either."

Suddenly I stopped in mid sentence for Daddy, has just put his hand to my face to silence me. He then pointed to some bushes across the meadow. There was something but I couldn't really see what it was. The next thing I heard was the crack of his rifle and what was in the bushes started to run, staggered and then fell. We went running. The deer had fallen head over heels.

Its head particularly, hidden under its body the rest in the bush. Daddy pushed the carcass with his rifle. Nothing moved. He shoved it with his foot, still nothing. He reached down and moved the beautiful, antlerless head, it was a Doe, and Daddy had a problem.

Not only was it no longer Deer Season, Doe's were strictly against the law. But Daddy was not about to leave it. The worst part was we were in his car, not his truck. We couldn't just tie it on the hood and drive down the highway. It wasn't going to fit in the backseat. Eventually there we were moving down the road with the Doe tucked in under the front hood of the car with the motor.

Sad but true, Daddy said:

"We have to get it home somehow".

During the spring and summer we would plant flowers around his house. Dad had about ten acres of land with a huge garden area. He was always trying out some new kind of seeds, sometimes he never even knew what it was supposed to be. About once a week we would have to go to the Nursery and see what new seeds were in. Then just plant the seeds and watch to see what came of them. There were times that nothing ever came up, and there were times that it was something very good.

The best reason I enjoyed going to my Dad's house is, that while I was there, I felt I was among people that really Cared and Loved me, for me. When I was at "home" I didn't experience feelings like I did when I was at my Dad's, never certain if it was for the reason that I was here because of the affair or what, other than I didn't experience Love like that. Or if it was for the simple reason that there were so many of us, and Mom and Papa just didn't know how to give love to all the children equally.

Therefore while I was with my Dad I had no worries. In addition there was never anything that I ever desired or wanted. My Dad would at all times make sure that I had the all the fine things that I could ever want or need. All right, yes I will be the first to say that I was one spoiled child growing up. My Mom, Papa and Dad did whatsoever they possibly could to give me *Things*, as I was growing up.

Other than that I had a pretty simple childhood growing up. I just went to school, and came home, never actually had friends come over, nor did I go over to friend's houses or anything similar to that. I would just ride my bicycle up and down the street and visit the neighborhood families.

During the summer months when I was not at my Dad's house, I would sit out front and wait on the postman. I would walk and talk with him or her as they would deliver the mail to our block; we had the type of mailboxes that were up by the front door, so the Postman would have to walk door to door to deliver the mail.

Neighbors

Benitez Family

As a child, particularly because I was the baby by so many years, I wondered about our street looking for playmates. Since this was a small street in an older section of town, there were no other children, so my friends became many of the Seniors who lived there. I was precocious, and fun loving, and somewhat of a tomboy. Falling down and scraped knees and elbows were always visible. One couple down the block, were my special friends and they comforted me when I would get hurt. To stop the tears and get me to laugh when I fell down for one hundred and first time, they use to say that because I was so bubbly my blood didn't ooze out, it fizzed.

Russell – lived next door

There was an elderly man that lived next door and he was a POW from WWII. His name was Russell. Russell and I would sit down out in his front yard and have picnics and just chatter about different things.

"Hey my little Acorn head" his favorite words of endearment for me.

"What are you up to today?"

"Hey Old Man", my way of teasing back,

"I was just serving lunch here on the grass"

"Momma gave me some cookies and said to share them with someone special, but I can't find anyone like that".

We sat and laughed at my joke and then shared some Oreo's. I ate the cookies and he ate the insides, because I do not like the middle stuff. It used to look so yucky, him trying to eat cookies around the plug of tobacco he almost always had in his mouth.

He at all times, had stories to tell about his days in the Military and his days from when he was a Prisoner of War. He never had any children, subsequently he always treated me like the child he never had.

During the school year when it came time for Report Cards he would always ask to see my report card.

"Annie isn't today Report card time?"

"Yes Russell why do you ask?"

"Well, having been in the Navy I like things that are Red, White and Blue, and I wanted to see how much Red is on that White and Blue Report card of yours."

"There's no Red I did very good."

He would also have something for me, for having Good grades, sometimes it would be a dollar for everything from an A-B, or he would buy me a special gift.

We would always just sit down there in his front yard and we would just gaze at the leaves as they would fall down from the trees, at the same time we would be having us a picnic. There would be times that we would take his dogs for a walk, he had four large dogs and the dogs loved going on walks.

Russell passed away a couple of years ago. Within a couple of weeks after his passing I received a phone call from a Lawyer to come into his office that we needed to talk. I asked what about? That is when he told me that Russell …. had put me in his Will. Little did I know that every time I got my report card from school, and he would always ask to see it. He would put money into a savings account for me, as a Reward for making good grades. I never knew this until he passed away.

The Lawyer told me about the Savings Account surprised me that Russell had left me his house as well. I was around twenty two with all the responsibilities of providing for my children. I was overwhelmed by my change of fortune. The house sat right next door to my parent's house. You know this is the only secret that I never told my mom or anybody else. There was no way I could live next door to my family so I sold it. No one ever knew it was left to me.

Brother's and Sister's

Tony (oldest Brother)

One of my favorite siblings was Tony; he would take my spankings for me,

"Mom you can't hit her she's just a baby"

Mom replied "she needs disciple and someone's bottom is getting it", so Tony took my spankings for me.

Then there was a time that I remember, Tony had to go to work and he was supposed to be watching me, I was about seven or eight. He placed me in the kitchen cabinet and told me: "Do Not come out no matter what"

"Do not come out till I come back to get you". I said "ok"

So I sat there and then I started hearing voices. It was my Mom and some of my other brother's and sister's.

"Gayla, Ricardo have you seen little Annie?"

"No Mom don't know where she is"

Since she cannot get a hold of my brother at work, the next thing I hear is:

"Police this Mary at ...."

11

"I left my six year old daughter here with one of my sons, he's gone off to work and she's nowhere to be seen."

Moments later the police are at my house, and I can hear them talking.

"Mam, is she the type of child that would run off?"

"Would your son really leave her at home alone?"

In my mind all I could hear was my brother saying:

"STAY IN HERE do not come out No Matter What!"

After a while, despite the fact of what my brother, had told me I was getting worn-out, so I wrote a note and slipped it underneath the door, and asked if I could please come out, saying that I was frightened and hungry. I hoped that somebody walking by might notice it. Sure enough somebody did see it; one of the police officers saw it. They opened the door and asked how come I did not come out when I heard them talking?

And I told them that Tony had told me:

"Do not to come out No Matter What!"

After that came the million questions.

"Why were you in there?"

"How long have you been in there?"

"Where is your brother?"

So I told them what he had told me. "Do Not Come Out No Matter what!"

Boy did he get in trouble that night.

Cindy (oldest Sister)

Then there was the ever jealous Cindy who would lie about anything, and everything, to make me look bad. I remember one day (after I had been married to Mike and we were separated I had moved out) Cindy came by my place, to pick something up at my house that I had with the kids. She then left and went to our mothers to tell her that I had locked the children in the closet without their dinner.

Fortunately my cousin Jennifer was there babysitting because I needed to go out. Just then mother called wanting to know what was going on with her grandchildren. Mom had told me that Cindy had just come by there and that she had just left my place, where I had the kids locked in the closet and would not feed them.

I told my Mom "hold-on, talk to Jennifer"

I then handed the phone to Jennifer without saying a word to her.

She took the phone and said:

"Hello" and as she listened she was getting very angry.

"Aunt Mary I was here when Cindy came by, and when she was here, and still right now the kids are sitting at the table eating."

Jennifer went on to explain that Cindy's story was a complete lie. The kids were never locked in any closet at any time.

Jack

Brother Jack and truckin', I guess because music is such an important part of my life I often use words and music to describe events in my life. Even though Willie Nelson is not one of my favorite entertainers,

"On The Road Again"

Became one of my favorite songs. As I have indicated many times, my family was large and since I rarely felt like part of the family, any attention was welcomed.

My brother Jack brought something beautiful and adventurous into my life from the time I about twelve until about age sixteen. Jack drove a big rig, a diesel truck, and although it was strictly forbidden to carry passengers, I often was his traveling companion.

"Whoa!"

No one get any funny ideas. I was just experiencing seeing the country, and he had someone to talk to while trying to get through those long hauls. It wasn't during school times, and for me it was being part of the family. Later in life it made it easier for me to meet new people, and travel the road myself and not be afraid. It also gave me a great sense of direction.

Jack would pick up his rig at the terminal and head out. One of my other brothers and I would meet him somewhere down the road and I would hop in with my travel bag. We covered most of the USA, being gone sometimes a week at a time. While my classmates learned from books about geography, I experienced it firsthand.

Jamie

Depending on the time of my life, the fact that my brother Jamie was a Bull Rider was either very exciting, or "is he out of his mind."

The ensuing fact that at age nineteen, his was the body in the casket we all stood mourning over and cried about, it took all the thrill away.

Garth Brooks the singer, sings two songs about Rodeos and Bull Riders.

In *"The Beaches of Cheyenne"*. We hear about the thrills and excitement of being part of the Rodeo circuit we learn of the devastation of learning what happens when the Bull wins and crushes a loved one to death. In *"Rodeo"* they talk about the bulls and the blood, and the joy and the mud, and who wouldn't be attracted by adoration of a screaming crowd. I was only six when Brother Jamie lost his battle of the Bulls. Thirty plus Years later the scare is still there and open.

Jr. High School

Jr. High, Wow what a different place. Remember it was during this time that I found out the true story regarding my parents. I found out that my Mom had an affair with my natural Dad; they were together for about a year or so, anymore than that I can't ever seem to get out of them.

The way I found out about this was I overheard my Mom and Papa talking about me going to the other family's dinner that weekend. And my Papa did not want my Mom to go because he (my dad) would be there.

"He who" I thought.

So I just sat there listening, and that is when Mom and Papa started talking more and more about what had happened several years earlier, and that they were going to have to one day tell me the real story about everything. Well me being young and nosey, I popped in and said:

"What are you talking about?"

And that is when I got the whole story. Some days I wished I really never knew. Plus my Mom and my Natural Dad, still to this day, see each other at least once or twice a month, now just as friends.

My dad is always coming into town for something or another. My mom always knows when he is going to be in town, and they make it a point to see one another.

While in Jr High, the majority of all the children constantly made fun of me, the entire time for one thing or another. I despised Jr High. For one thing, I had extremely long hair, down passed my butt, and my Mom would by no means give me permission to cut it.

Consequently a number of the girls that sat behind me in class would take my pony tail and place it up in a twist and call me an old lady. Then there was PE Class, I hated the entire changing in front of everyone. At age eleven I was an overflowing "B" cup and as for the rest of the girls, the only "B" they knew was on their report card. As a result I would always get ill and have to go to the office for the duration of that time period.

So that I would not have to change in front of the other girls, or just even the thought of running made me feel sick. Everyone always made fun of the way I ran. First came two boobs, followed by two feet, Thank God I didn't have a big butt trailing behind, what a sight that would have been.

Subsequently the school nurse caught on to me. So I asked my Mom: "will you please write me a letter to get me out of PE?"

Well my Mom did one better than that; she got me a Doctor appointment so he might write me a note to get out of PE all together. Because, you see I developed early and all the girls would make fun of me for this reason. So, Yes my Dr wrote me a note so that I would not have to go to PE. He wrote: "Due to a Medical condition Annie will not be able to attend PE."

All the children would make up jokes about me like:
"Have you seen Annie's New shoes?"
"No"
"Well she hasn't either."
They would say because: "her boobs are sticking out so much she can't see them either."

My nickname in school was BB – Big Boobs.

I never used to wear make-up or fix my hair, I just combed my hair straight or I had it in a pony tail. In my final year in Jr High School, towards the last part of the school year, a Group of the girls that I had just started hanging around with cornered me; they said:

"We have determined, you need to start wearing make-up."

"We cannot permit you to go off to High School looking like this!"

The next thing I knew they had held me down and covered me in make-up. No one at home had ever talked to me, or helped me to put make-up on so I never wore it. Then they *cut* my hair. I had my hair in a ponytail that day; they just cut the ponytail and said:

"Now your Mom will have to let you go get a haircut."

Then I had to walk all the way home, because I had missed my ride home, and I cried all the way home, I just knew my parents were going to kill me. I got home and there was no one there, I am out of harm's way I thought, for the time being anyway. Well before I could get in the house and at least wash off the make-up, my Mom pulled around the corner and saw me. Well I just started crying even more.

The look on my Mom's face, I may perhaps never be able to explain. You know the look:

The look of Shock, and Horror, of what has *my* child went and done?

The only thing she could say was

"What have you went and done?"

I told her about what the girls did. That they cornered me and did it and what they said:

"We have determined you need to start wearing make-up."

"We cannot permit you to go off to High School looking like this!"

She demanded everyone's names and information, but I could not give that to her. The girls were just now beginning to

17

speak to me, so I was not going to do anything that was going to alter that.

Later that night my Mom took me to the beauty shop to get a cleaned up hair cut. So I went from sixty (60) inches of hair, to about four or five (4-5) inches of hair just like that. And it was so much easier to manage and to style.

While I was at home and growing up I never actually even had a Birthday Party, or anything like that (my birthday is Christmas Day) so no one would come any ways right!

Mom and Papa would make sure that at all times I had whatsoever I sought after. I had my own room while at home, where most of my other brother's and sister's had to share. I even had my own phone line, TV....

Sharing my Talents

I entered High School in September of 1983, and my Dad has just bought me an entire new wardrobe, to get High School started with. Mom and Papa bought me a new car. Well High School started off with a bang, new clothes, new car, and a new hairdo and now I am even wearing make-up. Within the first couple of weeks of school, when students were doing all the try-outs for all the different groups, theater, dance team, choir,… I found my place.

I started getting involved in Theater, choir, dance, and anything else I could come across to do. I was so thrilled we are having our first Play. I told my family about it, told them the dates and times and even got them all tickets.

The saddest thing was none of them even showed up. On every occasion that I had an event my family would not show up for any of them. There was always something else more important going on. After the play all the other childrens families came to tell them how proud they were of them, but no one from my family. Then the second concert came, same thing, no family there then the third, then the fourth,…… .

After awhile I just got used to it. Even to this day, my family does not come to any of my concerts or plays. Whenever my

Dad is in town and I have a play or concert he would come but he was the only one. I knew it was hard on him, since he lived so far away. Although I have eleven other brothers and sisters, most of them have never been to one of my plays or concerts.

Except one, he is the one that I am the closest to; he also feels at times like an outcast, I kept telling him that one day we are going to discover that he is really the product of an affair or something like that.

Then one day it happened, one of my sister-in-laws let it slip, we found out that my brother really was my nephew. One of my sisters had gotten pregnant when she was very young and could not handle the thought of being a mother, she was going to put him up for adoption, and that is when Mom and Papa decided that they were going to take custody of him, and they adopted him when he was only about two to three months old. To this day we don't know who his natural Father is.

I feel bad for him, having to grow-up not knowing who your Natural Father is. It is kind of like not knowing who you really are. There is an empty feeling there.

Incredible Opportunity

While I was in High School, throughout the summer months, I would go to New York City to The Juilliard School, for dance and music. My Mom did not like this at all. She wanted me to have nothing to do with the Entertainment Industry. I went back and forth about four to five times. I had even started instructing a number of classes during the time that I was there. I just wanted to pack up and move to New York and live there permanently. Right before I left New York City the last time I got to do a voice over for an animated film. It was so exciting, I met so many Awesome and remarkable people, and it was great.

A lot of hard work but ton's of Fun. I have made friendships that will last a lifetime and will ultimately change the course of my life's pathway.

It is currently the starting of my twelve grade year. In addition it is also time for me to leave New York City. Time to go back home and get prepared for my Senior Year. My flight home was late getting back into Dallas / Fort Worth arrived back in Dallas, late and I couldn't sleep, therefore I went out and sat on the porch that night, and this guy came over from the house two doors down.

He was living there in the house with a couple of other guy's.

He said: "I haven't seen you here before are you visiting?"

We talked for a short while; he was asking me about where I had been, and what I had been doing in New York. So we sat there and talked about, where I had been, and what I had been doing while in New York City.

His name was Mike. Mike was a little older than me, and was already out of school. He had just moved into the house down the street, a couple of months earlier, we went out a couple of times and it immediately went from there. One minute we were just acquaintances, the next thing we were talking about moving in with each other the next thing I knew we were talking about getting married.

Marriage to Mike while in High School

Within about six months we did get married. As usual nothing changed, with my family. Only one of my brothers came to the wedding ceremony. It was to be a small wedding; just family and close acquaintances. Well it was small alright, only one of my brothers, and Mike's, Mom, Dad and just a couple of his friends were there.

Everybody immediately thought I would not finish school, but nevertheless I did. Just a couple of months before we got married Mike decided he was going to join the Army, so while I was finishing my Senior year of school he would go off to boot camp. Before he left for boot camp, within the first couple of weeks of marriage, I found out that I was pregnant. Consequently the only thing that actually changed with school was that, I had to limit the number of the groups that I was in, like Dance or Theater.

My new friends thought it was cool to have a married and pregnant girlfriend within their grouping of friends. They were forever asking: "could we give you and the baby a Baby Shower or something?"

A lot of my friends had taken on the role of being aunts and uncles. Well April came and the baby was born, a Precious little girl. All my friends came to the hospital to see their New Niece. This made Mike very angry that they all came up to the hospital. And I slowly started losing friends one by one. Every time one of my friends would come to the hospital or to the house after I was at home, Mike would just be so rude to them that they started not coming around anymore.

By this time Mike found out that we were going to be moving to the "Army Training Center for the Infantry in Fort Ord, California"

Before I could go I was going to finish school, of course I went back to school two weeks following the birth, and finished school. I kept up with all my work, I even got to Graduate along with my class.

Move to California

It is now that time, for me to pack up and join Mike in California. He loved this because now he had me away from all my friends and family. We lived there on base, in base housing.

The first time Mike became the person I didn't know or understand was once we moved to California. Away from family and friends. There were moments of:

"I am the Man",

or "it's my house"

But it was only words. One evening after just hanging out, Mike walked over and grabbed me. I didn't understand and even said:

"Ow! That hurts, what are you doing".

Mike replied, "You're my wife and I can do whatever I like".

"So shut up bitch",

"It will feel good, and you will enjoy it".

I didn't and my fears grew. But at eighteen and very innocent I guess it was what a wife was supposed to do, so I did not know that else to do but submit.

Sex was excepted whenever he said: "Sex"

Sex was new to me but I had never been treated like this. Mike was my first partner and I had no way of knowing better.

There were times I was subjected to this type of humiliation, and in time a natural part of too many days and nights.

Every once in while we had intercourse, and what use to be a little pleasure became an ordeal for which I took because it was either that or to get slapped around.

During the California days Mike, also was a challenge to my return to College. I had taken more advantage of my High School year's academically than Mike. I also knew that without an education my future was limited. Mike has his family money and no need to advance himself beyond where he was. He also couldn't face the possibility of being put down because he wasn't the sharpest knife in the drawer. Each day's going to classes was an experience.

Every minute that wasn't His time, was supposed to be for cleaning, cooking, and meeting his needs. My studying was done during classes, and the development of my mind left to time driving, or in the shower, or when there was a desperate need for sleep. The worst part was the demeaning comments about:

"Women don't need an education;"

"Women are here to take care of the needs of their men, and have babies".

Mike's parents did not like the fact that he had joined the Army, let alone having their first and only grandbaby taken away from them, just a couple of months after she was born. The fact that we are living on the base. His parents even told us as long as we lived on base that they would not be coming out to visit us.

It was not so bad at first; everybody was very helpful in getting us all settled in. There would be times when he would have to go out in the field and train for days and weeks at a time.

I knew one time that Mike was going to have to be in the field for a month, so I made plans to go back home and visit family and friends while he was gone.

Once I got back to the base and Mike got back home, from being out on the field. That is when we started having problems. It was while he was gone for that month that something changed him. I am not sure what happened, or if I will ever find out what happened. But it was at that time, when he started getting very controlling, and did not want me to do anything at all what so ever.

360 - The Day it all Started

Today is the Three hundred and sixtieth day that we were married; I woke up and walked down the hall, brushed my teeth, then slowly walked toward the kitchen. This was another morning just like the other Three hundred and fifty-nine mornings before it. Dear God if only number Three hundred and sixtieth would have been the same.

Day Three hundred and sixty became day one (1) of the physical abuse that ripped my body apart, left me with seventy-five to a hundred different scars, and the remnants of thousands of stitches all over my body.

Like Ed McMahan became a regular on the Johnny Carson Show, I became a regular at the local hospital and Emergency Room.

So following Graduation along with the baby and moving to California, I knew my New York City days were over. Mike by no means wanted me to do anything with my performance career, or anything that had anything to do with Dance or Theater. He did not like other people looking at me at all. He would even point out some one that was looking at me; he would want to know:

"Do you know them?"

No matter the answer it would anger him.

We lived in California for his full term, and Thankfully he did not re-enlist. Both of our families were very happy that we were moving back home to Texas. Mike's family was so excited they had already gone out and found us a house and everything. Things did not get any better once we got home. Mike still did not want me to do anything. He did not want me going to visit my family, friends, or anything like that. He did not even want me to work, he only wanted me at home and if I was at home he knew where I was at, and if he needed anything I would be there to get it for him.

He worked for his Dad at the family business. His Dad owned quite a few businesses' all over the area, and he would just work with one of them here and there. That would be the only way that Mike could work, because he would have to have off every Friday – Sunday. So even if I did want to work, there would not be anybody outside the family business that I would be capable of working for, and have these days off.

So consequently I would stay at home throughout the week, but however every Friday – Sunday we would pack up, and head out to go off to our River house which was about two – three hours away. Somewhere, where He could live out his dream, and Barefoot Water Ski whenever he wanted to. Each and every weekend no matter the weather conditions we would have to pack up on Thursday as well as drive down on Thursday Night so that we were at the River on Friday Morning. That is when the water is the best is first thing in the morning. Smooth, Calm water if we woke up and the water was like a mirror we were going to have a good day, otherwise if the water had ripples the rest of the day would have ripples as well. There would be anywhere from thirty to fifty of us, on most all weekends.

I did learn how to water-ski; however, I did not get to do a great deal of it. The reason being I had to pull him instead; it was all about the stillness and the calmness of the water. It was not about pulling anybody else, it was at all times what he considered necessary. If the waters were not calm and at a standstill, we were pulled up on the shoreline waiting for the water to get calm. So as long as we had calm water for him to barefoot water ski I knew that everything else was going to be ok.

Everything was going pretty good, till one day I was doing laundry when I found something in his jeans. It was a baggie of Cocaine. I asked him about my finding it. As a result of that we got into a terrible disagreement, and he told me that he had been doing it for a long time, and that I could not prevent him from doing it. He also enlightened me that he was also selling it as well.

I thought about this for awhile, and then I told him:

"You are going to have to discontinue using, and selling, or the baby and I were going to have to leave."

He got extraordinarily irritated and as a consequence of that he threw me through our back glass sliding door. I got all cut up, and we set off in the direction of the hospital. If that was not enough, I had a total of one hundred and thirty four stitches on my forearm, face, and the top of my head. At the time he pushed me I put my arms up in front of my face, and with that it was the only thing that prevented my face from getting all cut up.

That was followed by my finding out, that Mike was also smoking and selling pot.

Mike came into the kitchen. Apparently he was having a particularly difficult day; someone forgot to tell him how wonderful he was. Definitely not me or if I did, I said the wrong words. Mike just walked up to me and popped me with the back of his hand.

"You are a worthless piece of shit, why are you in my life?"

I said: "You know I can change that."

He turned and walked away and soon returned.

He looked crazy and angry and I don't know what to call it. He grabbed me, and said,

"Possessive little devil!" and threw me across the room.

"I control your life and I can take it away whenever I choose and no one can do anything about it".

This time I was truly angry. I was going to leave him; we talked about it along with telling his parents of what our purpose was, and that we were going to separate.

1ˢᵗ Try at Leaving

The thought and consideration of separation with the possibility of a divorce was unheard of in this family. They completely could not handle that, not within their family,

"You are not" they both said

"No one in this family has ever had a divorce"

"And we are going to keep it that way"

"We are not going to be the first of this family to have one going through a Divorce".

So they took care of the baby and sent us off to their Condo up in Colorado for a week for us to attempt to work things out. They were not at this point aware of his drug use. And with that we headed out for the week.

The first day we were there I took snow ski lessons. Mike went skiing by himself. The following day he decides I'm good enough, and he wanted me to go to the top of the mountain with him, so we headed for the top of the mountain, to what they called one of the effortless routes.

Consequently we set off to the top of the mountain and it was just beautiful. At the top of the peak we went to a restaurant and had a little something to eat first. After that it was the moment to start the journey to go down the mountain. He told me to just tag along right behind him, and for me to do what I was taught yesterday. I thought okay, and then we were on our way straightforward and down the mountain. From out of nowhere there was a white out, it started snowing so hard, and the flakes were so large, that I could not distinguish anything.

He says again: "just follow along behind me,"

"If we are capable of getting to the next landing there was a different restaurant where we could possibly just hang around there for a short time".

Well that would have been very well, if he would have stayed on the uncomplicated slopes, but, NO he refused and we had to go down and over to a Black Slope (hard) I was following him, but I could not slow down, then from out of nowhere; there was a tree in front of me. I ran right into the tree, and broke my goggles, ski pole, and twisted my skis all up.

Did he stop to help or lend a hand?

No!

I could barely move about, I was trying to just make some slow progress crawling down the mountain. Then shortly a Red Cross snow mobile came.

He said: "Somebody going up on the ski lift saw what happened, and sent us down to find you."

Once they got me on the snow mobile, and we were on our way to the bottom, the snow had lightened up slightly. Along with that it was looking pleasant once again.

"And where was Mike?"

Well he went back up to ski down for a second time. I never found him at the bottom so the resort called me a taxi to go to the hospital to get my injuries looked at. So I went to the hospital and had to get my leg casted, it was broke in two places, I called Mike from the hospital to come and get me and take me back to the Condo. He told me:

"Catch a taxi"

"As I'm going to go and sit in the Hot Tub for a while!"

33

The rest of the trip I just stayed inside the Condo and he went skiing every day. Finally the day came that we get to go home.

We got back home and his parents are like:

"Okay~!"

"Everything should be back the way it's supposed to be?"

Even though I had told them about him leaving me on the top of the mountain to find my own way down with a broken leg.

Mike's mom told me: "sometimes we just have to turn our heads and look the other way"

"You are home now, and that is the main thing"

"Now we have to work on keeping you happy"

A couple of months went by, not much of a change. Mike really likes to play golf, I have played around with it a little, after all I did have nine other brothers, and we went to the golf course about once a week to play a round of Golf. All was going good till I had started getting better and I had better scores than him. Then one day I had several holes in one. Then, from out of nowhere, in just a split second, he took a BIG swing; hit me right in the nose. It busted it all up, there was blood all over the place. He took me to the Club House; where the staff there convinced him that I needed to go to the hospital. Once at the hospital they found out that I did not fracture the nose bone, it was just cut up bad and they stitched it all up, it only required about nine stitches.

Now for a short while everything was going better, until one day I found more drugs, while I was cleaning the house. Afterwards we got into another huge argument, over all of his drug use. I was in the middle of cooking dinner. When he reached for the pot that I had on the stove, he intended on throwing it at me. I saw it coming and moved, but not fast enough, and therefore it burnt my legs. Once again I had to go to the hospital; it had burnt my legs, as well as a cut which required twenty-three stitches down my leg.

I remember telling Mike's mom about the Drugs after I got out of the hospital.

She said: "you know we must stand behind our men and support them in what they do"

I thought:

"Did she not just hear what I said?"

So I asked her "did you hear what I just said?"

"Mike, *your* son is selling and doing DRUGS!"

She said "yes I heard you"

"And like I said" "we must stand behind our men no matter what"

"All men have their faults"

"We just have to learn to accept them and live with them."

Mike wasn't big on, family members coming to visit. It was not much of a problem, for my family since they very rarely even came out to our house anyway. On the account of when they did come out Mike was so rude to them, they just started not even coming out. Since Mike was an only child, his only family was his Mom and Dad, and his parents were always gone out of town traveling, more than they were at home.

His family was at the same time as horrifically bad as mine, in that when they would discover that we desired something, they would go out and get it, before we would have the opportunity to go and get it ourselves.

For instant when we got married, despite the fact that I was still in High School, we moved into a small apartment. His parents would not accept the thought of it, and bought us a house. Then when we moved to California they just made it a rent house.

Then when I had Elizabeth I got an 8ct Diamond ring. Along with that they bought a very large quantity of items for the baby and for us. They had to bring all the gifts to the hospital; for they couldn't wait till we got home. They had to make sure everyone saw how much they had bought , so they brought it all up to the hospital; it took Mike two truckloads to get everything home prior to being able to take me and the baby home.

Consequently I went from being spoiled by one family, to another one that was even worse. Since his family owned a number of businesses in town, money was not an issue; also they were on all the city council boards.

Things immediately got considerably worse. If I didn't perform everything accurately, just the way Mike wanted it done, if I didn't do it immediately, just the way he required it to be done, then I would get the crap beat out of me. As a result I stayed at home a lot; I didn't feel like anybody seeing me all black and blue or with stitches, or whatever the injury of the moment might be.

There was one occasion while we were driving down the highway, while Mike had been drinking. He had just finished a beer and he took it and threw it out the passenger window on the side which I was sitting. Not only did my window happen to be closed, but as the beer bottle hit the truck window, it broke both the bottle and the window, and glass went all over the place.

Once more it was my fault since I should have had my window down so it would not have ever happened. Back to the hospital again to get patched up.

Of course I got cut, but no stitches this time, "Yeah!"

This time the Doctor's asked for me to talk with a Social Worker, because my file was getting pretty thick.

The Social Worker asked so many questions:

"Is someone at home doing harm to you?"

"Are you afraid to go home?"

"Can you tell me how you keep getting hurt?"

"I see this is the third time this month that you have been here!"

I just told her "that I just need to be more careful"

I have countless scars, several you are able to distinguish, along with even more you cannot see and then there are the scars that are on the inside, which I will never forget.

As my abilities expanded, and the people around me became were more dependent on my decision making, the worse the relationship with Mike became. My strengths made him more insecure, thus the more often and more severe the beatings became. Insults became slaps and punches, leading to my fingers and legs being scared and broken, to my face being slammed and pushed through windows and against mirrors. There was a sick sort of upside. I got to know and make friends with some of the nicest Hospital Staff and Resident Doctors.

My family was ushered into a misguided view of me. All the accidents were my fault according to Mike, or that is what he taught them.

"If Annie was more careful she would not have fallen down the steps."

"If Annie would look where she was going she wouldn't have walked through the glass patio door."

"When you are cooking you have to be careful,"

"If not your hand gets caught in the flame of the stove, and hot food spills all over your Back and Head."

Despite the fact that, there was a great deal of physical abuse, there was also all the emotional abuse. I frequently thought that possibly after a while Mike would change. Boy was I mistaken regarding that one; from time to time I sincerely believe that it got worse. Since not every single moment of my time and focus was on him. We had a little bundle of joy in addition now, to take care of as well to be concerned with. It just got worse.

Is it safe to take a Shower?

Have you ever dropped a hot charcoal on your leg?

How about sticking the skewer from the rotisserie from the barbecue in your foot.

How about sitting on a large screw drive?

Not even close to being shot.

On one occasion when I was preparing to go in and take a shower, I was sitting on the edge of the tub, about that time Mike walked in and said something to me, I looked up, and there he stands pointing a gun at me. My heart did several serious flip flops I immediately knew I was fixing to be shot.

He said:

"Oh you didn't even consider I was going to use it did you?"

He turned and walked away, and I went back to getting ready to take a shower.

When all of a sudden I felt it.

It hurt so badly!

He had shot me in the back. Oh it hurt so dreadfully bad.

The bullet entered by backside and a burning erupted and I thought I was about to die. He then strutted out of the house.

I then just laid there and waited. I thought I was going to die, and my baby was out with my Mother. So I just laid there and waited.

Death was becoming my main focus, and survival was protection. I was pretty sure that I was going to die before my time.

The "when" was the only question?

Mike's, family's connections would keep him safe and out of jail. A year later I would learn how true that really was.

The neighbors heard the shot and called 911.

After Mike realized that he had shot me, and that the neighbors had called 911, while we were waiting on the EMT's.

He just kept saying:

"We will tell them that I was just cleaning the gun."

"That's what we will tell them I was just cleaning the gun"

The EMT's and the police are now there and getting me all ready to go to the hospital, Mike tells them:

"I was just cleaning the gun and it went off".

Well the EMT's are now putting me in the Ambulance and Mike tells them:

"I am going to follow in my truck, but can I talk to Annie first?"

He got in the Ambulance and says:

"We are going to just tell them that I was cleaning the gun when it went off." "If you tell them anything other than that I will make you pay!"

The entire time we were at the hospital he just kept saying:

"I was just trying to clean it, that is what we will tell them right"

And then he would repeat it:

"I was just trying to clean it, that is what we will tell them right"!

Well now the Social Worker really had questions. It had only been two weeks since I was in last. They even made me stay in the hospital for a couple of days. Whenever anyone would ask what happened, he would just tell them the story of cleaning the gun.

You know his parents never came to the hospital to visit during this time. But once I got home Mike's mom came over and told me:

"You need to start paying more attention to Mike"

"Or I can see things getting worse."

I thought "how much worse could it get?"

She said: "Mike Sr. has done some of the same things to me"

"You just have to learn to turn you head and not make him angry."

A while later, here I am getting ready to take a shower, and there is a snake in the bathtub. I screamed and Mike came in there just a laughing, he knew why I was screaming and came in to get it. He had found it out in the back yard in the garden area, in addition to it he wanted to keep it, therefore he didn't know where else to deposit it at the moment.

So therefore if I was not getting hot water thrown on me, or getting cut up from this or the other, I was being tormented by other things, and being scared out of my wits.

The Unexpected

Then all of a sudden and totally unanticipated, something even worse happened, I found out that I was pregnant for a second time. This time the baby was due in Oct. As a result I was going to have to go throughout the summer months pregnant. It made pregnancy hard, difficult, and complicated, imagine going thru the summer, going to the river during the one-hundred degree days pregnant as well as having to pull him skiing. It was a battle every time he sought after going and it was just Hot plus I was miserable the entire time. It had even gotten to the point that I almost about lost the baby. It was at that time we found out that I was carrying twin boys.

This frustrated Mike even further; he said that now I wouldn't have time to keep him up, you know cooking, cleaning…..

Mike was a pain in the ass. Also my back, both legs, two arms, my boobies, stomach, and of cause my face. I have scars on both cheeks, my chin, and above and below both eyes. Most of the time it was from punches, or things thrown at me. Sometimes things I was thrown through. Then there was his cigarettes. I was his favorite ashtray. An arm, in my hand, and then there was the time he used my eye. You would like to think that something like a cigarette in the eye was only an accident, but the only accident

I ever related to Mike was his being born. So as a result of that, every time Mike would be smoking one of his joints, (marijuana cigarettes) he would take it and push it down on my arms, until I would scream. Now I have scars on my arms from where he burned me with his cigarettes, they are not as visible as they once were, but I know they are there.

I have had surgery to fix my eye. It took a total of nine different eye surgeries to fix that one. In the long run it was worth every one of them. I will now be able to see my children grow up.

Well the day came and we went to the hospital and the boys were born, everything was going pretty good for a short time. Oh and by the way along with having the twins we got new furniture, not for the purpose that we needed it, or anything. Just because that way when friends would come over we could let them know:

"This is what Mike's family gave us for a Baby gift."

Then for a couple of months everything was going ok, then from out of now where the old Mike was back and it started all over again with the yelling and the beatings, I told Mike about my intentions that I was going to have to leave I could not handle it to any further extent. That is when he pushed me and I fell and I had torn a bunch of the ligaments in my leg, so as a result to that I had to have to undergo knee surgery two times to repair everything.

2nd Try at Leaving

After the knee surgery we once again told his parents, that we were going to have to separate, and they once again sent us away for a week, this time to Cancun, with the anticipation for us to work things out.

He even turned around and was, sweet and charming some of the time while we were there. We were having a Wonderful time, till one day when we went out on a day yacht cruise and swam among the sharks and sea turtles.

While swimming among the sea turtles they started trying to consume my hair. At this time my hair was very long, (I had let it grow back out) and I was told that the turtles may have thought that it was seaweed floating along the top of the water. Mike just stood there and laughed, whereas everybody else, besides him is trying to help me get free from the turtles.

I had decided that was enough, after we got home I was leaving. I did not say anything about it while we were there. I just went along with the rest of the week, just watching, along with listening.

You see Mike had gotten addicted to Drugs big time, in addition to drinking a lot, I was worn-out from being his human punching bag.

It was at that point in my life in which I said:

"That I have got to leave, because we are not doing either one of us any good."

Therefore, after the trip we took, I attempted to work things out. So that once we were back home, I started the process of looking for a place for me and the children to move. I establish a place for us, along with knowing that his parents were going to be out of town for awhile, I told Mike that I was leaving. As a result he got extremely angry; I was not only frightened for me but also for the children.

I told him: "we were not doing each other any good at all, and one of us was going to get seriously hurt."

The Worse Night Ever

This would be the night that everything would change. At that instant I gathered up enough of the children things along with some of my clothes that we would need for a couple of days. By this time the children were two years and the twins were six months. The children and I left, as I was driving down the highway, all of a sudden and unexpected Mike passed me and motioned for me to:

"Pull over."

I could tell that he was intoxicated along with most likely had taken some of his other drugs, that he was doing at that time.

I just kept driving; me in my Camaro, and Mike drove a Chevrolet long bed pickup. Well it was at this instant that the rest of my life had changed. As soon as I did not pull over, he pulled up alongside me and told me once more to

"Pull over."

We are on the highway mind you. At that moment he pulls up in front of me on the highway and throws his truck into reverse.

Now I sit looking at what was once the windshield of my car. A strange view of what was the rear undercarriage of Mike's truck. I don't know which I believed less, the fact I was still alive, or that after all the other horrible experiences Mike had done to me that he would try to kill his children as well.

His truck rolled up and over my car. The babies were all in the rear seat. Elizabeth was sitting behind me, the twins Jackson and Jacob six months, were in the center sit, and behind the passenger sit, I was pinned in the vehicle.

I was in total amazement that he had done this. The EMT's got there very quickly, and they starting getting everyone out of the car when they realized that the children were in the rear seat of the car. That is when we realized that Mike had driven over the passenger side of the car, and killed one of the twins. The police got there and placed him under arrest for DWI and Manslaughter.

As circumstances would have it, for a change Mike got everything he deserved. Since his parents were out of town, their best friend the Judge was not made available to him. He had to stay the night in jail. He was in there for only three days. When his parents got back in town they got him out, immediately. Added to that his parents got together with their friend the Judge, and he got Mike off everything. The only good was, that despite the fact that Mike was in jail, and with everything else that was going on, I got all of the childrens as well as most my belongings packed up and moved out to our own place.

I'm still able to hear some of our friends at the moment saying:

"I cannot believe you are leaving him, you've got it all: Money, a Huge House, plus everything that anybody could possibly ever desire."

For a split second I stopped and thought about that, and then I told them that all the wealth, possessions and materials things were not important. I was worn-out, by way of being his punching bag, on every occasion when he would get drunk, or at when he was on his drugs.

That if I stayed it would before long merely only get worse, and furthermore I was not going to be around for a next time.

"I have already lost one child, how much more did I have to lose?"

After the Accident

After Mike's parents got back in town, Mike told his Father about the historically event, telling him about the accident.

Mike's Father said "I better make some phone calls".

His first call was to Brendon, golfing buddy and the town Judge.

Mike Sr. said to Brendon said: "I'm coming over"

Mike Sr. told Brendon: "we need to put a stop to this, my son's not going to any jail."

Brendon said: "Mike" "She's saying you tried to kill her and the babies."

"Jackson is dead," "Elizabeth and Jacob were injured, not severely."

"Annie was badly cut."

Brendon told Mike Sr.: "Mike don't get ahead of yourself."

"Let me get the Police reports."

"I'll meet you at Sims Park in a couple of hours."

"I'll call you with a time."

The accident happened shortly before midnight and Mike only sat in jail for two days.

Brendon called for Mike, and they met at the Park.

"The Police reports are a "he said she said".

"She is giving more details," "but we are lucky," Mike keeps moaning "it was an accident; I didn't mean to hurt the kids".

Judge (Brendon) made their plans. Mike would say that he thought she was running away with his kids and he just wanted to stop her and get her to come home.

"I got past her and noticed she had stopped back a ways."

"I put the truck in reverse, there was no place to turn around, and I started backing up."

"I just didn't judge my speed; I was so scared that I was going to lose my kids."

"The next thing I knew was the impact,"

"I was on top of her car."

"If she didn't do this, it never would have happened."

"One of my other Judge friends will dismiss all charges and declare the incident and accident."

When you have "money and friends" "in high places, there are no jail cells," "even when a child has only had the chance to experience six months of life."

The good was his Mom finally came to the realization that we were not going to be together. She would not accept or otherwise even consider the thought of her son being on drugs. In reality she did not want to face that fact (that did not happen till many, many years later). She told me with stipulations; if I would just leave and not tell anybody about what was going on, she would purchase a house, and a new car on behalf of the children and me.

I let her purchase it all, so that the children and I could get on with beginning our personal lives over. One other part of the agreement was that her husband, Mike Sr., was to know nothing of this. The main reason and my motivation to permit her to do this, was at the time I was not working, and it would help get us started.

The best thing is, that the two babies and I now had and safe secure place to live. There was no more loud screaming or yelling going on. Now just quiet and calm days and nights.

This happened so early in the childrens lives that they do not remember any of it. They do not even remember their Dad and I being married, or living in the same house. So as to that, with that purpose in mind, it was a true Blessing.

Mike and I were married for only about three years; and it was the hardest three years that I know of, it was a very, very, very abusive relationship. It was so abusive that I would have to go to the hospital at least once a week for most of the marriage.

Marriage to Mike is Over

Consequently the next step was for us to put the house on the market that we lived in together. We did and it sold for $688 thousand. We split it

and we each got in excess of $300 thousand. Later the courts established that he had not been paying any of his child support. Then he lost part of his share and the courts gave it to me. As a result I went and opened up investment accounts for the children for when they got older.

Wow everything is beginning to look up.

My next step was for me to decide what I was going to do. I couldn't just sit around the house and do nothing. The only predicament with that was, I would require to come across something that I could perform from home. I that I did not wish to place the children in day care, they had been through enough as it was. I immediately started the process of investigating something to do at home. As a result of that I started doing bookkeeping on behalf of quite a few different large companies, as well as a number of individual's. This would keep me busy and productive while being there for my children.

Everything was going good once more, till I got the call from my legal representative. He told me that Mike had just gotten the privileges to be able to see the children and they scheduled it for every other weekend.

Well the first occasion he was to pick them up on a Friday afternoon he was to bring them home on Sunday Evening. All was fine and good except it got to be 6 PM, no children. I called to reach him, and no response. At 8 PM no children, I called for a second time, and he answered.

He said: "I'm just going to keep them till in the morning,"

"I will just take Elizabeth to school in the morning, and bring Jacob home after that I drop her off at school"

I said: "good enough".

Not a great deal I could say at that point, he had them and I had no clue of where he was living, I would have had to of contacted my lawyer or else the police, and the children did not need that.

That Monday morning I went to the school, the children were to have a small little play intended for the parents, I made a promise to myself that once I had children and they had something going on, I was going to be there at least ninety-five percent of the time. If you remember, that when I was growing up I knew what it felt like for my parents not to be present. I did not desire for my children to experience that.

Much to my disappointment Elizabeth was not in attendance. As I sat there waiting to see her, I learned from the teacher that she was not present. The teacher came over to me to and asked:

"Where is Elizabeth?"

"Is she at home under the weather or what?"

I told her:

"Her Dad was supposed to bring her to school this morning."

I left there extremely angry, in addition, not real confident at this point what to believe. I went home and called him to discover why Elizabeth was not at school!

He said: "we over slept,"

"As a result we just stayed at home,"

"It's no big deal she's merely in Kindergarten, she will be okay."

I also remember another occasion, he picked them up, and we had the understanding that he was to bring them home on the following Sunday Evening. He did not; he had one of his buddy's bring them home. At about that time I answered the door Jacob had a huge bandage around his head. As soon as I questioned it, his friend said:

"No big deal, Mike was carrying Jacob on top of his shoulders, and he walked into a ceiling fan and cut his head."

He still has an awful big scare on top of his forehead to this day. Just about every time Mike picked up the children they were either behind schedule coming home (a day or two every now and then) or else they would have gotten hurt somehow.

Meeting David

Well it is currently 1989 – and I am in need of something additional to accomplish. The children are getting older, both are now in school.

So as a result I opened a Gift Shop –

"Gifts for Everyone"

It was great. In addition the children were able to go along with me to hang out there throughout the day, furthermore at the time, they were both in school, it will provide me with something to accomplish each day. Success in business also provided a new circle of amazing friends.

Also within this year I started dating all over again. A lot of them were just jerks similar to Mike. I was not going to do that for a second time. This went on for about a year. One day I was introduced to a man named David. He was a little older, and with three older children. He was all right. We went out a couple of times however there were no sparks, we talked about it as well. We determined to just be friends.

Easter was approaching, and at that time I was helping with a non-profit group, for an Easter social get-together that was approaching. I asked just about every single person I knew if they would wear the bunny costume, No Luck. Consequently I finally asked David if he would wear it.

He said: "yes I will wear it" - "with one stipulation that you will go out with me."

I said: "okay"

Good enough, the next thing I was to decide where we were going to go, so that I could tell all my friends to be there. I did not desire to go by myself. We enjoyed being in each other's company, but I did not want him getting any ideas. I even told him,

"I will go out with you but I am not getting into a permanent relationship any time soon."

David replied "I don't understand, nothing could have been that bad"

I told him: "maybe someday I will throw you down the steps, or push your face through a glass door."

"Perhaps when I take out a gun and swear I'm not going to shoot you"

"And then, then you feel the pain of being shot in the back after all,"

"You'll come to understand"

"Or maybe I can just back over your car and try to kill you,"

"O how about I put your kids in the car with you".

David looked confused "people don't do that."

I told him "Here are the scars that confirm the story."

"Let me take off my make-up, and maybe someday I'll take off my clothes and you can see the remnants of over one hundred stitches."

"Next time you come up behind me and I jump three feet off the ground or I just stand there screaming in fear,"

"You'll get the idea."

Finally he admitted that although he didn't really understand, he would try to learn. We talked and discussed everything that had happened while I was in the relationship with Mike, and why I was not interested in anything right at this moment. He said he understood, and furthermore he said he was fine with it.

But time and understanding were just words to David. He lived in his own Pollyanna world and the next thing out of his mouth was:

"You are going to make a Beautiful December Bride."

I told him: "Oh no I'm not; I'm not going there for awhile."

A couple of months went by and we were getting to be really good friends. Nothing any further than that, we just enjoyed going out also having conversation regarding everything that was going on.

Teddy Bear Park – More time was spent with my children, Elizabeth and Jackson. The kids really liked him because he gave into their every whim. Elizabeth asked David for a new Disney doll, he didn't know what she meant and arrived at the house one day with a Mickey Mouse, Minnie Mouse, and a Donald Duck doll. Jackson screamed when there was nothing for him. David ran out and came back with a package of a dozen Matchbox cars. Not exactly what a two year old should be playing with. But he did take them to Teddy Bear Park, walking along, and singing the song "Teddy Bear Picnic", and watching all the people that were dressed up like Teddy Bears.

Well he stuck around, and a couple of months shortly afterwards we started dating more, and more. More months went by; we were still talking along with going out.

Deshawn

One morning I had a knock on my front door at about 5 a.m. I was awakened and walked to the front door to find out who it was. At that instant the door swung open, it knocked me down. There stood a large African American male, he had just busted down my door and came in. It was at this point in time that he raped me.

He finally left. It was a long while before I was able to call the police. They came right away; in addition to them coming I then asked them, if they would call David at work. David came immediately without delay. He stayed with me at the hospital through all of the examination and the waiting for x-ray's. The guy had hit me in the head and I had a pretty good size knot on top of my head.

In addition to all the questions.....

"What he looked like?"

"What was he wearing?"

"Did you notice if he had any scars?"

"Had you ever seen this man before?"...

In conclusion I finally got to go back home, David had somebody go over and fix the door. Luckily the children were with their Dad, so they were not there during this whole ordeal, and knew nothing about what had just happened.

Once that was finally over and a couple of days went by, the police department called me to come down and give them another description of what the man looked like. A couple of days later the police called me again to come down to see if I may perhaps pick him out of a line up.

Yes of course he was there and it was like reliving the whole thing all over for a second time. At that instant I felt him break down the door, and I was raped all over yet again. Weeks then months went by. Eventually it was time for court. At this point I found out that I was pregnant, by means of the rapist, yes I am now pregnant with the rapist's baby.

It was at this point that David said:

"Enough of this friend stuff we need to get married".

"You cannot have this newborn in addition to going through all of this court stuff by yourself."

As a result David and I talked in regards to getting married, and within a couple of weeks after that we got married. David moved into my house since it was paid for, and he was living in a small apartment.

Weeks along with months go by with many court dates. At last the long trial and court dates were over and Deshawn (the rapist) is departing to the penitentiary for about ten years. He knows that I am pregnant and expecting with his baby.

His wife was so sweet and charming. I met her during the trail, and I talked to her off and on. She was beside herself, trying to understand why Deshawn, could have done this. The blessing was that he confessed so as a result there was not a long drawn out, time-consuming court battle.

Once again my life is beginning to give the impression of looking up once more. Until one day while I am at the store shopping and I am about six to seven months pregnant, here comes someone from out of nowhere, somebody just accidently ran their shopping basket into my stomach. The impact was so firm it caused me to go into pre-labor. I was rushed to the hospital, where shortly thereafter I did have a miscarriage and lost the baby.

Months went by, and the loss of an additional baby was very hard to accept, even under the circumstance of the way it was conceived. I had many thoughts about Jackson the baby I had lost in the car wreck. I felt like it was necessary to go and tell Deshawn. So I contacted my lawyer and he was able to get me a pass to be able to go and see Deshawn. He actually felt sad on my behalf; I could tell he was actually taking it hard. This was a different man; this was not the same man that a year ago had broken into my house and raped me.

Being an all and forgiving person, following that first visit I went back about a month afterwards. I would go at least once a month to see and visit with Deshawn. Until the day he got out. He got early because of good conduct. No there was absolutely no attraction, just the attainment and bond of having lost a child. To this day there is part of me that calls him friend and a deep down hatred of what he did to me.

In time, he got out of jail and went to the seminary to become a youth pastor. It did take him lots of time; it did not come about overnight. At first the Seminary did not want to accept him to attend because of his past history, but in time they found out that he in actuality did changed. As a result they agreed to giving him a crack at it. I remember when Deshawn called me and told me he was going in this direction. I was so extremely excited for him. We stayed in contact all the time while he was going to seminar.

His wife would call me along with keeping me updated on how he was doing; he took several various courses at one time, so that he could finish earlier than he was expected to. He would complete two years worth of work during one single year, and of course I was in attendance on his behalf on his Graduation Day.

Even better than that, when Deshawn got out of seminar, a church immediately contacted him to be there youth pastor. He went and had a very long discussion with them, and they want him, he gets the job. He tells them that he cannot take the position until Annie comes in, and talks to the entire congregation and tells everybody her story.

Deshawn tells them:

"It would be to your advantage,"

"And it should come from Annie not me,"

"And that it would provide you with a clearer, and more complete picture of where I come from."

He explained that he could not possibly accept the position till after that. The senior pastor called me, telling me what Deshawn had told him; concerning him taking the position.

All was left pending on when I could get there, and telling the church my explanation of the situation. I asked the Pastor:

"Did Deshawn tell you anything in relation to my story?"

He said: "No, but on other hand I am guessing that it is extremely significant if Deshawn won't even consider the position until you come and talk to the church."

I was floored, so I agreed to go and tell my story. We talked about a date and got it all settled about when I would go there and recount the story.

The church was about six hours away. The day came and boy was I nervous, I had not talked to anybody concerning what had happened, other than very close friends, and the police.

It was a Sunday Night service, and the place was jam-packed. I got up and started telling my story about the events of everything that happened, my door getting busted down at 5 AM, getting raped, and even getting pregnant with his baby, him going to prison, then me going to the prison and visiting him and everything else, without saying any names.

Also, including the fact, that we have become really good friends, because we both forgave each other. Then followed after gaining the strength to speak, I told by telling them that person that I am talking about was Deshawn. The look of shock on their faces.

However at the same time they genuinely appreciated the fact that Deshawn wanted them to know. Also the fact that he asked me to tell the story, and by not having Deshawn telling the story, meant so much more to them.

They also respected the fact that Deshawn wanted them to know before he accepted the position as the youth pastor. Yes some of the youth were there that night, and every one of them, went and gave him and me a hug and a pat on the back.

Several months later I was asked to, at my church, to give my testimony.

I thought about it and said: "yes."

The next thing I had to find out was when this was going to take place. So I could call Deshawn, and ask him to be there. He said:

"I will be there, and so will my family"

So the day came, Deshawn and his family came in town a day early. The day came and I was so nervous, for the reason that, only my closest friends knew about everything. For this occasion, unlike the one that I told at Deshawn's church, I have been asked to tell my complete story.

My days with Mike and everything that went along with that, and my children did not even know about some of the things that I have been asked to talk about. Like at this time my son had no idea that he was a twin. I had always felt he was too young to comprehend, neither of them knew why their Dad and I were not together.

That was the blessing as I told you previously; they were so young that they don't remember all the beatings and the weekly hospital visits. So for that reason I sat them down prior to that Sunday and told them the whole story. They both said that it helped them to understand a lot more, and my son said that it helped him to understand the emptiness that he had been feeling.

Deshawn showed up that Sunday morning, and I think he was more uncomfortable than I was.

I said to him "Deshawn you have no reason to be nervous here, I am the one that has to talk".

He said "I know but I am the one you will be talking about. This is your church and all your acquaintances",

"Where they already know and love you."

"You have known these people for quite some time and they are very protective of you."

"When you came to my church you knew none of them and I had nothing to lose."

"I was prepared to leave if I had to."

"When your friends hear what you have to say,"

"Then find out that I am here,"

I stopped him right there, and told him: "trust me my friends are going to love you, just as I do"

"Just by you being here is going to mean a lot to them, and the fact that you brought your family."

He said "OK" and we sat down and were waiting for service to start, and as some of my friends started coming in, I would introduce them to Deshawn and his family. They would welcome him with open arms.

Deshawn's comment was "just wait until after service."

I told him "OK" so after service was over, so many people came up to me and Deshawn and told us how proud they were of us. If he was a friend of Annie's he was a friend of theirs, the past is the past, we must all move on.

So then after church a group of us went to lunch, before Deshawn and his family had to head back home, and we had another great time together. It also served to teach the children to understand forgiveness.

Deshawn and I are still good friends. As of a matter of fact I have been to Deshawn's church several time's for different events. Deshawn asked me to come and help his church with a program they were going to be doing. He wanted me to be one of the performers. So I went there a couple of times a year for this, that, or the other.

The church is growing very rapidly, and they are even looking to add on or to move to a new location. Where they are currently there really is not sufficient room to add on like they need to. Deshawn is now celebrating his Tenth year at the church. They have grown so much. I went there for his Tenth Anniversary it was Great to see him and his family again. A number of the now college children, that were Jr High or High School students when I first went down were there and they remembered me, they came and gave me a big hug.

I have met a lot of them over the years. It was nice to see them again and all grown up. They all just love Deshawn. I was in the town where he now lives, just the other day with a friend that knew a little bit on the subject of what had happened, I asked him if while we were in the same town if we could look up Deshawn. Well we did and then we made the arrangements with Deshawn to go and see him the next day, and what a Wonderful visit we had. He is still at the same church, after ten years they have grown a great deal larger.

It was funny; Deshawn and I talked the night prior to me coming in to see him, and about us coming to see him at the new location. William (a friend that you will get to know later) and I got up that morning and got ready to drive over to see Deshawn. I was so nervous, William had only heard about Deshawn, and about just a little bit of what had happened. So I did not know how he was going to take it. But the visit was great. Deshawn showed us all around the new location.

Then we went to his office where he still had the same secretary that he has had since day one. She is a very sweet lady, a little crazy, but great fun to be around. Every time I went there we would go out, and go and do something, shopping, eating out, to just riding around town.

Well after we walked around the new place, we went to Deshawn's office; it was too funny, I thought she was going to fall out of her chair before she could get up. Deshawn had failed to mention to her that I was coming in, and she was so excited she could hardly get up. She grabbed a hold of me and was just so excited; I looked over my shoulder at Deshawn and William.

I asked Deshawn: "you didn't tell her I was coming did you?"

He said "Nope I wanted her to be surprised!"

That she was. Then she just walked passed Deshawn and shoved his shoulder, and said:

"Next time you better tell me, so I am a little more prepared,"

"She even brought a friend with her, and here I am acting like a fool in front of him"

Breast Cancer

Shortly after I lost the baby I found out that I had breast cancer, I found it early, it was in stage II. It was contained in the breast tissue, in the lymph nodes under the arm. So I had – Breast Conserving Surgery / it removes only the part of the breast that is closely surrounding the tissue and the cancer tumor.

The treatment schedule for chemotherapy depended on what they found. I did both a Chemotherapy drug in a pill form and injected intravenously. Chemotherapy was given in cycles, with days or weeks off between treatments. This cycling allows the body a chance to recover between treatments.

An entire course of chemotherapy generally lasts three to six months, again depending on the drugs used. I had a surgical procedure to insert a device called a port-a-cath under the skin of my chest. This device remained in place for the next six months of treatment and it allows the drugs to be administered without a new IV being put in at each visit.

I went in once a week for six months; each visit would lasts from one to six hours, not all of which involve drug administration. It would all depend on my blood count for that day. Before I could have treatment I would have blood work to see what the different blood counts were.

I had a good friend that would go in with me and we would just sit there and visit or we would just read a book or watch television, while I was having my treatments. I never really got sick with all the nausea.

I did lose my hair, and after having *Long* hair almost all my life that was about the hardest part. So I got to the point that I really loved hats, I liked hats prior to but no one wears them any longer.

There was more of me to love also. Chemo will do that to you. I went from a size Ten to a size Twenty-four.

The one thing I tried more than anything was to maintain my days as normal as possible throughout my treatment. I worked in addition to doing a majority of the tasks that I normally did. I remember once somebody told me that it didn't seem that I had a hard time during treatment. I really did have an "easy" time compared to most other people, but I told my friends that it wasn't as uncomplicated as I had made it seem.

I just really did not want everyone to know what was going on, and how bad I really felt. It goes back to my days with Mike – "Just Grin and Bare It." "Always keep a Happy Face"

So I don't want you to think that I had set the example that it was doable without too much life interruption, but hope that I didn't make it seem too easy for those who may require treatment and have a harder time.

Attitude makes a lot of the difference.

Also during this time I had breast reduction surgery. From those days in Junior High, they just kept growing.

I was quite large in the breast area. I do believe that this part of the surgery hurt the worse than any of it. I went from a bra size of GGG to an EE. There are still times now that I wish that I would have gone smaller. But there is no way I am going to go through that pain again.

Marriage to David

David and I got married shortly after the rape, and I found out that I was pregnant by Deshawn. We can both honestly tell you, that we may have gotten married, but neither of us loved the other, like one should in order to get married. I remember him telling me one time:

"Maybe we will fall in love over time".

He was very sweet and he had three older boys of his own from a previous marriage. They did not like me at all; they thought that I was too young for their Dad. We never told them why we got married; we never told anyone that the pregnancy was from the rape. Everyone just thought that David and I got pregnant. When I had the miscarriage it saved the need to explain how David and I conceived a child with African American features.

Then David and I bought a house with the purpose of fixing it up. We were to make the repairs it needed then to put it on the market. During this time we were living it. Each day as soon as David got home, we would work on the house.

One day I had been out earlier out picking blackberries with my Aunt. As a result of that, that night after David got home we were working around the house. While outside in the backyard where the house along with where the fireplace met, there was an exceptionally large crack.

David gave me a container of spray foam installation to spray inside there. Well I was not be familiar with it, and did not know that it was going to expand in addition to even coming out. I attempted to shove it back up inside with my hands. As soon as I started pushing it back up inside there, David says something to me and at that moment in time I immediately pause with my hand still pushing it in.

Followed by, yes you guessed it; my hand is currently trapped in there, in the crack stuck between the house and the fireplace. Well David tried to get my hand out, except it was not effective. As a result he called 911. Plus it was an excellent approach to meeting every one of our new neighbors.

Once the EMT's were present, subsequently so were all of our new neighbors, we had barely been living there a couple of weeks. The EMT's said that they had some substance that would dissolve away the foam installation. It was acetone? It set my hands on a fire. Most of the pain and damage resulted because I had been picking blackberries earlier that day and my hands were all messed up from the thorns. Consequently it burned something horrible.

A couple of years later after all the repairs were done, I was ready to build a new house and move. It just seemed the house was getting to small so we built a little larger. I did not want a house that needed any repairs on it; I really did not want to go through that again. So we put the house on the market and it sold right away. The new house was not completeed so we put everything in storage and live in a hotel for about a month. At this time David's boys did not come over a great deal, they always thought that they got in the way. Also they thought that the house was too small for all of us, which was the reason that we got a larger place.

We hoped that they would come and see their Dad more frequently. Well I was wrong, regarding that one. Still to this day the only occasion they come around is when they need something or it is a good time for them.

Kid's Talk

My Children grew up in several different atmospheres. They became very adaptable and to this day never comment negatively about the past. From Five-Thousand square foot house of their birth to the two bedroom apartment that became home for the three of us and then when we added David, home was being together and the outside world imposed very little.

Elizabeth and Jacob were wonderful sister and brother. In the big house there were long large driveways to skate and bike on, a large pool and all kinds of swings and slides, even inside the house we had all kinds of toys. And when life could have gotten boring, there were always the Quarter Horses we raised and Elizabeth and Jacob learned and loved to ride.

Living in such an upscale neighborhood did not provide for a whole lot of children their age, but a never ending supply of Aunts, Uncles, and lots of additional Grandparents. Oh yes Grandparents, the kids did learn and develop sensitivities about their Grandparents. One set who had more time then they knew what to do with, and the others who shared everything with everybody. Elizabeth specially didn't like the restrictions at Mike's parent's house. The house was elegant, glass knickknacks all over the place, silky chairs, and white carpet. And antiques everywhere you looked.

"Momma", Jacob complained, "I got sores on my butt from having to sit in one spot" There were no refrigerator privileges and very few toys with which to entertain themselves with. Mike would not let them bring the things that would keep them amused because his Daddy didn't approve.

At Grandma Mary's it was the opposite end of the rainbow. The base of the family was Mexican American and families are precious and everyone watches out for everyone. The kids went out back to play or up and down the street where there were always the watchful eyes of neighbors. Kids played with toys, watched TV, and attacked the refrigerator with no holds barred. My mother often had negative comments about one thing or another, but there was always this little gleam in the corner of her eye for her grandchildren.

In the summer of '2000' Elizabeth now fourteen and Jacob twelve and I sat out on a great adventure. Just the three of us, David had other things to do.

"Mom how far is it to Victoria" asked Jacob.

"Mom, are we there yet?"

You should have seen the size of his eyes when I said:

"Only about Four more miles".

About Three miles later, past Corpus Christi and on to San Antonio, the mileage questions got fewer along with the "are we there yet."

Elizabeth was fascinated by the caves between San Marcos and Georgetown. She particularly liked an idea of leaving Jacob in the caves if he did not behave.

Elizabeth was a good student, liked school and got along with everyone. Well almost everyone. "Mrs. Annie this Mrs. Dedman the Principal at the school. We have had a problem with Elizabeth."

"What did she do?"

"I won't go into it on the phone, just come here immediately."

Out the door and into the car, zooming like the typical frantic mother. When I arrived they took me into the nurse's office. There sat Elizabeth with one of the better shiners I have ever seen. As the story goes, some girl was jealous of Elizabeth, because everyone liked her, so the other girl hauled off and punched Elizabeth.

Elizabeth was a lover not a fighter. She didn't fight back then, doesn't now.

Abuse starts again

David has started getting really depressed regarding the boys not ever coming over, and has started taking it out on me. Everything has changed once again. I couldn't do anything correctly; I can't do the laundry right, or cook right, even though I did run a pretty good successful Business, which showed a profit every month. At this point I still had my store, and it was showing a profit and paid for itself every month.

He would get to the point that he would make fun of everything that I did. So I stopped doing everything "cooking, cleaning – even when I would load the dishwasher – it was wrong" so I just let him do it all himself, after all I couldn't do anything correctly. After that I just wouldn't do anything at all while he was at home.

From then on I would not cook whenever he was around. He would even talk down to me in front of our friends.

He would state:

"Oh she can't cook; you don't want her to cook that!"

"She will mess it up!"

Keep in mind I grew up in a large family and as the baby spent years at my mother's side learning in the kitchen. Then there's my Papa who is a Chef in a very big restaurant. You think something might have rubbed off?

(Some of my favorite recipes are in the back of the book)

I remember on one occasion I was making potato salad. I peeled all the potatoes to place them in a pot on the stove-top to boil. After that David needed to leave and go to the store real quick and demanded I had to go with him. We went to the store and weren't gone for that long. He told me that the potatoes ought to be ready to mix them up. I drained them as well as completed putting everything in them. You know relish, onions, mayo…. Afterwards we tried a taste, ooooo my goodness, the potatoes were not thoroughly done!

And of course I got held responsible on behalf of it. So David deposited the whole thing back into the pot along with turning the burner down on low temperature to attempt to cook the potatoes a little more, of course the potato salad was by now already, all mixed up. Well that was a huge error. It burned up the entire potato salad, so of course I got the held responsible for another time.

After that I would just start cooking stuff and messing it up so that he would have something to laugh as well as talk about.

Whenever he was not around I would cook for just the children and me, and make sure that there was nothing extra left over, and if there was I would throw it away. I love to cook however, on the occasions I would make an effort to cook when he was at home. He would constantly make me second guess how much of this or that I have put in, and sometimes I would even wind up either not putting in the right amount, in or too much. He thinks he is just the greatest cook and that everybody only wants what he makes.

Times we would go out with our friends and they would be talking about something that had happened or something that they did. David would have already done it and done it better. No matter what the conversation, he would know all about it, or so he would assume. It would get old, there would be times when we were out with friends and he would say oh we were just talking about doing that. We hadn't even thought about it, or "oh we have done that?"

We've really never gone on any trips together. All we do is work and go home and that was the best part. Monday – Friday David would work 3 PM -11 PM. I still had my store and my hours were Monday- Saturday 9 AM -6 PM. So the only time we had together was some on Saturday nights. Every now and then he would also work Saturday's and some Sunday's. That was the best thing for both of us. If we were in each other's company anymore than that I am not sure we might have killed one another.

We are good friends just not a good married couple. So I am sure you are thinking so why are you still married? Why haven't we separated or gotten a divorce? Trust me it crosses my mind each day several times a day, however, I made a promise to myself that I was not going to put my children through all that.

They had already been through enough. So consequently my plan at this time is to just maintain what I have and keep putting money in my savings, and watch my investments. Once both of my children are either married or have moved out, that is when I will be moving out as well. I know it will be awhile.

Within the year I will move out and get my own place. I will have the house or whatever house we are in up for sale and we will be going our separate ways. At this time we are looking at a couple more years. So it does give me time to plan and get things in order, as far as finances and investments are concerned. I'm not much concerned about that part of it since David really does not know what I am worth. I have kept all that hush-hush, because when we got married, remember we were not in it for the love, so I never knew how far we were going to go, so I kept all my other investment matters in a separate bank account and the statements go to a PO Box.

The next Move

A couple more years have gone by, and things have only gotten worse. The children and I even moved out for awhile. We moved in with a friend of mine, I was planning on just going to a hotel for awhile, and they said:

"No you are not" and for us to just move in with them for awhile.

They also had a fairly large house, and most of the time we never even saw one another. We would leave notes in the kitchen on the counter so that we would know what each other was doing. We stayed there for about a month or so, but it was getting hard on the children. So we moved back home, and that is when I knew I would have to wait for them to grow up and be on their own or get married before I moved out and went on with my life.

So a little while later I thought:

"Sell this house, and build another house a little larger again, and maybe we could make it so David could have his own room,"

Because right now he sleeps on the sofa. We have a guest room but he won't sleep in there. He knows he would have to keep it cleaned up, because here lately we have had friends come in town every now and then, and they stay in the guest room. If he started staying in there he would have to keep it cleaned up. Sleeping on the sofa, all he would have to do is get a blanket or sheet.

So we started talking about selling the house, and I started looking at house plans. Then one night a huge hail storm come thru town, with very high winds, and it messed up the roof something terrible. The house plans got placed on hold for awhile.

Then it got put on hold even longer, after we got the new roof put on, I was out in the backyard walking around barefooted. Then all of a sudden I step on one of those roofing nails.

So now I am wondering when was the last time that I had a Tetanus shot. I called the Doctor's office and they did not have it on record for any time recently, so they said to be on the safe side come on in and get one. Then the next day I went back to the Dr because where I had gotten the shot at in my arm was extremely painful.

He told me to put ice and heat on it, for the rest of the day. Well the next day it hurt even worse. That following night I had a ladies dinner to attend that evening, so I was trying to ignore it, but it just got worse. While at the dinner I called my Doctor and he told me to come to his office and he would meet me there. Luckily one of the ladies said:

"I will go with you."

Red, White – I'm Blue

Wow here we go again;

I have been in remission from breast cancer for about eleven years now. I guess it was time for something new now to come about. Once I got to the Doctor he said it looks like the shot has crystallized in your arm.

So he numbed my arm and opened it up. The medicine had crystallized in my arm, it looked just like rock salt coming out of my arm. So he said we need to do a blood test, because I have only seen this take place in just a small number of other patient cases.

He said we will have the results within a couple of days. Within a couple of days he called me and told me, that I needed to come in so that we could talk. Well you know as well as I do when a Doctor calls and says you need to come in, it is never good news. I tried to get David to go in with me, but he had other plans, so I went in by myself.

We sat there and talked about the results for a short time, and then he told me I had Lupus. At that time I had no idea what Lupus was. So he sat there with me and we just talked about it for awhile.

Lupus is an autoimmune disease that can affect various parts of the body, including the skin, joints, heart, lungs, blood, kidneys and brain. Normally the body's immune system makes proteins called antibodies, to protect the body against viruses, bacteria, and other foreign materials. These foreign materials are called antigens.

In an autoimmune disorder like lupus, the immune system cannot tell the difference between foreign substances and its own cells and tissues. The immune system then makes antibodies directed against itself. These antibodies -- called "auto-antibodies" (auto means 'self') -- cause inflammation, pain and damage in various parts of the body

My Dr told me that I should attend a Lupus support meeting, he found one that was coming up, and then he told me I needed to go to it, so that I could find out more about Lupus.

I went to a meeting, and then said: "Oh No Way~!"

"This is not for me at all."

The only thing the ladies in this group talked about was how sick they were and that they could not do anything. This was not for me, I went out and found a book that was a huge help, and got a lot more information from the book, than I did from this group.

"Living with Lupus / All the knowledge you need to Help yourself" - by: Sheldon Paul Blau, M.D. with Dodi Schulyz

A couple of years have now gone by and my Doctor has just asked me if I wanted to go on a Medical Research Trip? With him and some of his other Doctor friends.

I asked him: "get me additional information and I would consider it."

To consider it I will have to either sell my store or close it.

That was just what I did I sold the store. Then started getting prepared to go on the trip. As days went by I would gain more information and then I found out that I would have to most likely be gone anywhere from two – six months.

That part scared me; I could not accept that I could possibly be gone from my children that long. They were not capable of staying at home unaccompanied at night; they were still too young for that.

Then one of my cousins called me and asked if they might be able to stay with me for awhile. They were in the middle of having a house built and their house had sold within days and they needed a place to stay. They had no idea that I was getting prepared to go out of town for a short time. We met up and talked about, and they agreed to stay at the house and watch the children for me while I was gone. It worked out great, because that they are both retired.

So it worked out great given the fact that David still worked nights, my cousins needed a place to stay, and I needed someone to stay at the house and watch the children for a short time.

Medical Trip

Well I went on the trip, on May 12, 1999 - my Mom took me to the airport to catch a plane to New York City. That is where I was to go to get connected with the people that were going to be doing the testing.

As I got off the plane in New York City I saw a gentleman holding a sign with my name on it. So I went over to him to let him know that I was Annie. Afterwards we went to obtain my luggage, simply to discover that they was not there, we waited for a short time. Then the airline rep told us to go on to the hotel and if they found it, they would get it to me, mean while they gave me a cash voucher so that I could go and get what I required for the night.

Now we are on our way to the hotel "Marriott Financial Center". When I got to the hotel there was a very nice Jamaican Man (bellman) on hand waiting outside.

He said: "You have got to be Annie B?"

I said: "Yes"

I was almost afraid to say yes. He then tells me "there are a couple of people inside waiting on your arrival." With that I went in and I meet the people there from the testing center. They give me my room key and told me to go up to my room and freshen up, then come on down for dinner, then they would introduce me to the rest of the group.

Everyone was so nice and so helpful. Well I went back down for dinner, to find out that I was not the only one here for the testing, there were about twenty of us. There were ladies from all over the place New Zealand, South Africa, Switzerland, Japan,....

We were told we could do whatever we wanted to tonight, but to have our luggage packed and ready to go at 6 AM in the morning. That we were going to Boston for the day.

So one of the other ladies and I went for a walk along the Harbor right outside our hotel. It was so beautiful; we could get a glimpse the Statue of Liberty from there, and she was all lit up. We walked for awhile then we all went back to our rooms to get prepared and organized for the next day. Once we got back I was told that they had just dropped off my luggage in my room.

In the morning, on our way out, we are taking a tour of New York City, our bus driver was driving all through the city, and showing us the city, Hudson River, Queens, Time Square, ...

Then we got on the highway and were headed to Boston. We arrived at our hotel in Boston, we all went to dinner, and while talking to some of the ladies here, it turns out that some of them are just like the ones from the support group back in Texas.

They feel that they have Lupus and they can't do anything. (It's really sad). After dinner I wanted to go out and see the city, one of the ladies went with me. We walked for awhile then I saw the opening for the subway. I told her let's go down and take a ride on the subway, I've never rode the subway before. She did not desire to have any part of that; well I finally talked her in to going.

While we were riding we were talking about where everybody was from, and how we all got to this point, and there was a gentleman riding close by, and he asked me:

"You have got to be from Texas?"

I said: "yes,"

He asked me to just talk to him; he just wanted to hear me talk.

He said: "I like to listen to people, talk that are from Texas."

Then after that when we got off the subway, and one of his friends was there, and they were getting ready to go to Texas for some concert.

He said: "Wow do they all talk like you there in Texas?"

They were very sweet and caught Kathy and I a horse and buggy to take us back to our hotel; they said that it would be too far for us to walk. So Kathy and I rode back to the hotel in the horse and buggy carriage and saw more of the city while we were riding along.

Today we went to the hospital in Boston for some tests. We will have more days of testing here as well. Today they have taken a lot of blood, and they have also taken several tissue samples. The Staff are all so sweet and treating us Wonderful.

The good thing is we are getting educated a lot in relation to Lupus, and some of the ladies are not as down on themselves as they were when we first got here.

Later that day we went out shopping, and one of the ladies bought something, and the next thing I hear is:

"Annie come here!"

One of the ladies had bought something for $2.89. She was bewildered, they wanted her to pay $3.13 (sales tax) where she was from they did not include sales tax. And she was trying to figure out what she had done wrong. From then on they would inform me how confusing our currency was, that ours was all the identical color, and identical size, and that their money is all different sizes and all different colors, and in their country they have no coins just bills.

We have just gotten word that one of the ladies here just got a phone call for her husband is about to pass away. He was sick with spinal cancer prior to her leaving. Her family wanted her to have these test done, she is from Australia, her husband and her family told her she could not come home yet, that she needed to stay and finish the testing first.

I talked with one of her daughters on the phone, and she told me:

"That if her dad did pass prior to her getting home, that they are not going to tell her till she gets home."

She said: "that they will have the funeral and everything if he indeed passes prior to her coming home.

I asked: "well what if she calls and wants to talk to him while she is away?" The daughter told me: "Not to be concerned, he hasn't been capable of talking for awhile for his voice is too weak"

I just thought - Wow!

Well we are now going to pack up and head to Washington DC for our next stop. And our bus driver has just asked us:

"OK who here is collecting rocks?"

We just all looked at him, he said "because some of the luggage is beginning to weigh a ton."

I told him:

"Well you do have a bus full of women, and you have been letting us go shopping."

"And furthermore, every appointment we go on they present us with stuff, like bags, shirts…."

So he said:

"OK here is what we are going to do when we get to Washington DC,"

"I'm going to get everybody a container, and everything that you are not going to need till you get home, like the stuff you have bought to take back home or anything that the different hospitals have given you, you can put in that container."

"That way we are not unloading belongings that you in really don't need on a daily basis."

We returned back to our hotel in New York City, where we would stay about another two or three days before we went back home. The entire trip was so meaningful.

It was great, to meet so many awesome people, we have already all swapped e-mails and phone numbers. The entire trip was a little long; we were out for only about six weeks.

Yes the ladies husband did pass away and no they did not call and tell her. They were even trying to get her to go on a cruise before she came home, just so she could take a break from all the testing before she went home. She did not go on the cruise; she told them:

"No she just wanted to go home."

I talked with the daughter for a second time, and she said:

"That he did pass away, and they had already had the memorial service and everything."

"That they just had a very small funeral with just the family,"

I asked her:

"What are you going to do when your Mom gets home?"

She said that they are going to plan another Memorial Service, for the rest of the Family and for their Friends, once her mother got home.

One of my fondest memories of the friends I made on the trip is that it was so hilarious because on every occasion when we would all got together one of us would say something that the other as no clue of what it was. So our main topic while on the road were the different words that we say verses the words they say:

Their words – Our Words	Their words – Our Words
Loo – Bathroom	Lolly – Candy you suck on
Foum – Bench	Potato Crisp – Potato Chips
Boerewors – Country Sausage	Biltong – Beef Jerky
Peak Cap – Baseball Cap	Hair Slide – Barrette

4x4 Cab – Van	Serviette – Napkin
Napkin – Baby Diaper	Dummy – Pacifier
Dungarees – Overalls	Anarak – Raincoat
Handbag – Purse	Purse – Wallet
Boot – Trunk	Bakkie – Truck
Biscuit – Cookie	Crackers – Dry biscuit
Sweets – Candy	Takkies – Sneakers
Mother Chick – Chaperone (Annie B)	
Robots – Traffic Lights	Braaivleis – Barbecue
Indicators – Blinkers	Goeie More – Good Morning
Molo – Morning	Basin – Sink

Well today is the day that we get to go home, in addition to that the Good News is that we did discover a drug that would help us to feel better. Not a cure, but nevertheless a pill that would assist with the pain.

Home from Medical Trip

Consequently I am now at home, and getting back into the swing of things, trying to catch up with everybody and everything that went on while

I was gone. So many things have changed in the short amount of time that I was gone. The children have grown and they look great.

A couple of months after getting back in town I was at home and now nothing to do, since prior to leaving I sold my store, cause we did not know how long I would be gone. Prior to David and I getting married I would perform with a Band, so I called them up to see if they were looking for anybody new to join them and if they were, I would like to be considered.

They were like "Yes" "we would love to have you back."

Fortunately everything that they had coming up was local, so I would not have to start right off the bat traveling, I could stay at home with the children and they could even go to the different concerts as well. The children loved going to the concerts.

Followed by that I even started Home Schooling the children so when we did get to the point of traveling they would still be able to go. This went on for about a year and a half.

Then I had to leave the group, David was getting actually quite ugly. My Lupus started acting up again, and the children were getting older and they really desired to start getting their lives together, and they were missing their friends. So I agreed to do one last tour of concerts, and the children were going to stay here at home and start back to school. We talked about it; it was going to be about a four to six week tour. It was to be a Wonderful tour, we were to start and finish in New York City. At this time I had about three weeks to get ready.

Last Tour Trip

(July 25), - Well I just got back to New York City and it feels like I never left, we are staying at the same hotel that I stayed at before when I was here earlier with the Medical Organization, the "Marriott Financial Center".

Our bus pulled up and it was so cool looking, it was painted jet black, with a scene from Cinderella – the pumpkin carriage being pulled by the horses. The bus even has two bathrooms and about ten TV's and the chairs were great, they will unfold out into a very nice and comfortable bed. The TV's are set up to where we can all be watching something different if we want to.

(July 28) We did a very small last minute concert at our hotel the first night we were there in New York City and the next morning the bus picked us up and we headed for Mystic, Connecticut.

It was a very cute little town, we had dinner there with some of the stage guy's and we laughed so much that we did not believe that we were going to be capable to even sing. We finished everything up there, and after that loaded back up on the bus, so that we could head on into Boston, where we would be staying for three to four nights.

When I was in Boston the year earlier I was not able to go and see the entire city. So during the day we took a city tour, they have so many really cool looking brownstone buildings, and a lot of truly neat stores. We did a small concert in the Cheers Bar there, now that was cool.

(Aug 9) From here we are headed off to Canada, we went to Quebec City Canada, wow it is so nice here, cold but very nice, so our first stop of course is to go shopping on behalf of some warm clothes. Since it was in July at the time when we left the last thing on our minds was a sweater or anything along that line.

It is very much a French town here, and people are standing on the sidewalks playing instruments or painting and selling them right there. Everywhere we go they are speaking French, even when I attempt to make a call out, the operator is even talking in French. I was trying to make a call on a land line because I just found out my cell phone was not working, I didn't have International on it, boy did that change as soon as I was able to get a call out, I got a hold of my Mom and asked her to call my cell phone provider and have International added to my phone so I could call and talk to the children.

(Aug 26) The hotel in which we are staying was Wonderful; it is right on the river. We are now getting ready to leave here and now headed to Montreal, Ottawa, then to Toronto We stayed at each of these for about three to five days.

On the way to one of the spots we stopped off at a Place called 1,000 Islands, and took a boat cruise tour, it was so Cold, the Houses there were so cool looking. It is right on the border of the USA and Canada. And it is 1,000 Islands with homes on them; the 1,000 Islands are a chain of Islands, that stretch for about fifty miles. There really is one thousand eighthundred and sixty five (1865) in all, and range from forty square miles to smaller. To be considered an Island it must be above water level three hundred sixty five (365) days a year, and bigger than one square foot and support at least one tree or shrub.

We have now crossed the border to go back to the States. We are supposed to be doing some small concerts along the way back to New York City.

(Aug 30) Our first stop was in Washington DC. First we got to go on a tour thru the Capital and we had to go thru about five different check points to get in. While we were there we also got to go and see the Arlington Cemetery, along with the Internal Flame, at the Kennedy Memorial.

A couple of days later when we were getting prepared to leave the hotel, there the bellman came to my room to obtain my luggage, I opened the door and his pull cart was loaded up:

I told him: "I can wait on the next one"

He said: "Not a problem I can get it on top of here."

I looked at him and said: "there is no way you are going to get my luggage on top of all that you already have on there."

Well he grabbed it and tried to swing it up to the top, then he just put it back down, and asked:

"Do you have dead President in there?"

He said: "that is heavy."

"I told you it was not going to go up there."

So we agreed that I would wait on the next one.

(Sept 6) Next stop was to be New York City – till our bus broke down in a little town, in Lancaster, PA. So Joe called around and found us a place to stay for a couple of days. Fortunately we had a couple of days to spare. We stayed on an Amish Farm for a couple of days; it was very interesting, we walked the grounds along with talking with them about the way that they lived.

At mealtime it was great, it was just like it used to be many years ago at home. Everyone sitting down for dinner, and passing the food up and down the table, and there was so much of it. Then once we went to our rooms that was it, not a thing to do from this point but to go to bed, no phones, TV's or anything. It is like being back in the 1800's.

(Sept 9) Well our bus is currently fixed and we are headed back to New York City. Joe is on the phone trying to acquire tickets so that we may be able to go to a show tonight. It would be cool since we don't have any shows to do tonight we can go and see a show ourselves, just have a relaxing night. Joe did get us tickets we are going to the show River Dance. Our tickets were great we were in the pit!

On the way back to the hotel following the concert, we stopped off at a Deli, since it was late everything else was closed, and we had some of the finest sandwiches ever. Once back at our hotel, we were greeted by our favorite bellman Carlos.

He said "I haven't seen you in awhile,"

"I have been here every day"," have you not came out of your room?"

So I explained to him that we had been traveling for the past couple of months. And we are due to go back home in a day or two. The last couple of months have been great, I have just talked with the children and they sounded great.

(Day to go home) Well it is the morning we get to go home. We're going to all go down to the lobby at approximately 10:30 AM – 10:45 AM for a late breakfast, before the bus picks us up and takes us to the airport.

I'm up and taking a shower, when I hear this awful noise, and heard a bunch of commotion. "Yes it was the first plane hitting the Twin Towers." I looked out the window and there were people running all over the place. Then followed by that, about that time the second plane hit the second tower.

We were staying at the hotel "Marriott Financial Center" that sat right in the middle in front of the Twin Towers of the World Trade Center.

I remember hearing all the alarms going off in the hotel then I could hear everyone screaming to evacuate the building, I got dressed real fast and went down nineteen flights of stairs, because the elevators were jam-packed full, it was a mess. I really did not think that I was going to make it to the bottom. Everyone was screaming move, go faster, come on we have to get out of here.

Once I got to the bottom, I saw Carlos and he told me where the rest of my group was. We all got together and went out to catch our bus, when about that time a big piece of debris fell on our bus. And it was at that time we were told to start walking towards the Manhattan Bridge, and to go on the other side.

Everybody started running towards the Bridge, at that time even more debris started falling. This is when I got tripped and fell and got stepped on a number of times by other people. Several people in our group got hurt and were taken to different hospitals.

We were all separated. A day went by and I have not been able to get a hold of my family yet. We have all been trying to use our cell phone to call home except all the lines are tied up; we cannot get an open line because all the circuits are full of activity. Therefore it was about two or three days later before I was able to get a hold of my family and let them know that I was ok, that I had a broken leg, hand, and some burns on my face, we are still not certain how I got the burn, other than just the fall and perhaps sliding on the cement. The others as well had broken legs, hands, and cuts and scrapes.

We were all separated and taken to different hospitals, so we were not certain about one another for a day or so, till we were all able to get back together. Given that, there was no place for us to stay before the time for all of us to be able to go home, and I was the last one to be released from the hospital, everybody just camped out in my room. The hospital employees brought in several comfortable chairs for them to sit in. The chairs would also recline so that they could stretch out, with the purpose of they would have a place to sleep at nighttime.

The hospital employees were so sweet they did whatever they possibly could to make certain that we were all comfortable; they even allowed us, to use one of their cell phones once our batteries ran out to call home.

Then a couple of days afterwards as we were all getting prepared to leave the hospital. We were all in the hospital for about a week. I also remember that some of the AA employee's came to the hospital to stop in and see us and visit us, numerous times that week. They as well went and saw some of the others that were there, not just our group.

It did mean a lot to us for them to come and visit. They would always bring candy or something with them. Therefore, nowadays, every time I fly, I take a little present for the flight attendants, and let them know what a wonderful job they are doing. Maybe; one day I will run into some of the ones that came to the hospital to visit us.

The day prior to when we were to leave, I got a phone call from NBC News, and they asked if we would consider being interviewed on the Today Show. They wanted to talk to us before we headed back home. I informed the rest of the group, and we all talked about it and decided to do it. We told them we just had one dilemma, and that was we had no transportation to get there. They decided they would come and pick us up, then afterwards, make certain that we had transportation to the airport. So as a result they came to the hospital and picked us up, and just about all the hospital employees that had been helping and working with us came to tell us bye.

We went to the Studio and did the interview. Shortly after the interview, and talking with the staff at the station, they took us to the airport.

Everybody was so sweet and supportive, since a lot of us either had cast on, or were in a wheelchair. When we went out, there were six limos lined up to take us to the Studio then on to the airport. Everybody that was not familiar with us, were looking and trying to figure out who we were.

Now we are on our way to the airport, and when we got there, there was media all over the place, TV, radio, newspaper... at this time it has been about two weeks from the time 911 happened. Consequently we have to get to the airport five hours before time in order to even make our flight.

The good part is that we did not have any luggage; as a result we did not have to be concerned about all the security for getting our luggage checked. Since we lost everything that day, either at the hotel, or on the bus that we were getting ready to get on that got debris all over it.

Flight home after 911

We are now getting on our flight and there are sixteen of us returning back home to Texas. Everything was going Awesome. We left LGA @ 7PM on a non-stop flight from LGA to DFW. And at about 7:30 PM we were served beverages, it was at this time that everything changed. It was then that the lady sitting next to me flipped down her tray table to discover a note that said:

"The plane is going to blow up at 8:30 PM".

I at that time we showed the gentleman sitting next to us, who was an African American. He was sitting next to the aisle, and he turned white as a Ghost.

He then stopped the flight attendant, and she in return took the note up to the pilot. A short time later she came back to let us know that the pilot said:

"That we were going to make an Emergency Landing at Washington Dulls."

So at that time I asked her:

"Could I may possibly move and go and sit with my friends."

Because at that time I was not sitting with any of my friends, we were all separated and sitting all over the plane.

She said:

"Yes of course, however you cannot tell anybody what is going on".

Yea right~! I got up and went back to where several of my friends were sitting. There were two of them sitting together with a seat vacant in the middle of them. As I was walking towards them one of the other flight attendants approached me and asked:

"Is everything was okay."

I guess she could see it on my face. I just told her:

"I am going to sit among my friends."

I was telling Tom that I wanted to sit with them, and he thought I was messing with him. So he did not get up for me to sit down. Remember I have a cast on my leg and my arm. So I just climbed over him and sat down in the empty sit.

Tom realized that something was really wrong. At this point they have not made an announcement regarding what was going on. I told Tom and Mary what the lady had found and what the other flight attendant had told us. We then looked out our window and nearby there were two "F-16's" on both sides of us.

At about this time the pilot came on and told everybody what was taking place in addition to that, we were going to have to make an Emergency landing, and the pilot went through the whole speech of what to do, head between knees, brace yourself, and about the Emergency doors.

As soon as we landed they were telling the ladies no heels if you have on heels you must take them off, and that we could not take anything with us. Wow we are going to have to go down the slides, and over half of the group that I am with, is in no position to go sliding, down the slide, so the flight attendants made certain that there would be somebody to go down with us to help us. Plus the fact that we had to leave everything on board, no purses or any other of our carry-on's. Well I grabbed my cell phone and crammed it down inside my shirt. We landed hard and quickly, and at that time we immediately stopped right there out in the middle of the runway.

There was no taxiing to the gate or anything. One of the ladies within the passengers was one of the ladies who train's flight attendants for situations like this. She took charge of those Emergency doors. Well she might be little, however after seeing her in action with those doors and yelling at everybody, I will not get in her line of attack. We went down the slide, it was at this moment that I got messed up for a second time. As I told you earlier, when we had just left New York City, a couple of us in the group were still injured from the events of 911. Justin had burns on his arm, Mary had a broken arm, James had some stitches on his face, and I had a broken leg and hand.

Well we all started going down the slide, I got out the window, and Nancy (the flight attendant) yelled out to somebody that I was on my way down with a broken leg, and arm.

I will never forget the lady who was sitting next to me, as we went down the slide, There was a police officer down close at hand who said, he would assist her. Well she went down the slide and he did assist her alright. Instead of him helping her, he got right in front of the slide to make an effort to catch her. Well he caught her, she slide right into him and broke her other leg, and the police officer got hurt in the process. So once I landed at the bottom, I saw her wipe out the police officer, then I saw her trying to crawl away when the pilot and a fireman came over and picked her up and carried her off to the Ambulance.

While the EMT's were getting me ready to go to the hospital to get my other leg x-rayed, they put her in the Ambulance with me, we then shared an Ambulance and it was filling up with FBI, Fireman, and the Police. They were asking us questions regarding the note, and on the way to the hospital one of the officers said:

"I wonder what time zone they were writing this on?"

Fortunately one of my friends was capable of going with me to the hospital.

When we got to the hospital, News Media was all over the place. Well I now have a cast on both legs. They just got us a taxi to get back to the airport, to meet up with the rest of the group. I called the group, on the way to the airport because we knew some of them had gotten off with their phones. So we called them, that way we would know where to meet up with them.

Once we got to the airport, at about 1:00 AM, we met up with the rest of our group, to find out that they had been held up in a room to be questioned for most of the time. The airport had been evacuated, and the TV Media was all over the place, once again as well.

Well we were finally put on another plane around 3:00 AM to go home. We were not sure we wanted to get on the flight or not, you know following everything else that had been going on, this flight, 911 and all that went on with that. But it was the only means of getting home.

The flight was good and all, when we got home we had a bus on hand waiting for us to take us to meet up with our family. Of course the TV Media was present there again, you know because there was a group coming home from New York City and they are Survivors of 911, and now Survivors from a Bomb Threat on the plane from New York City.

The next couple of weeks were very trying, every time I turned around somebody sought after an interview. After I got home I found out that everybody had seen us all on the News, and for a number of them it was the first time that they heard, that we were okay. We are now all home, one day we were watching the news, and saw where a AA plane had crashed in New York City, and they did not know why, as we were watching the news about this crash one of the guy's said:

"Wow"

"Look at the flight number."

The flight number of the plane that had crashed was 587 and our flight number was 785, it was just backwards from our flight number. We just thought about it for awhile. That was just too weird.

Well finally as the weeks went by life has slowed down. Months have now gone by, and I finally got all the cast's off. Now I will just have weeks of Physical Therapy, but I will by no means ever forget that burning smell, or the loud crashing sounds.

I can be out doing something and I hear some type of loud boom or a loud crash and I jump. It is just like that day all over again, for a second time. I am extremely jumpy, like if somebody walks up behind me, and I don't have any idea that they are anywhere near, I jump or scream. There have been times they have scared me so bad that I just wheeled around and I have even hit them. Just because they have scared me. I don't mean to, it is just a protective reflex.

In addition showers are not the same any longer, because I was in the shower when I heard the first plane hit. If I am in the shower and hear a loud noise, it is similar to being there again. Even though all I heard was this loud booming crash, it was what came following that, the fire alarms and looking out the window and seeing people running all over the place.

I can be out and smell a house fire and it is no where around where I am except I can smell it. I remember one night just a while back I was at my aunt's house and I told her I smell a fire! She was like all right. Well I left there and went home and within about thirty minutes from her house I found the fire. That is just one smell that is going to stay with me.

Several of us from the group get together at least once a week, to talk about what all has happened. Now, it just months away from the One Year Anniversary, and we have just been asked to attend the One Year Anniversary,

"Oh wow go back there"

"Are you crazy?"

Well I guess we are, we have started making our plans to go back for the One Year Anniversary, at Madison Square Garden's.

I know that this is going to be hard, most likely one of the hardest things that I have done. One of the first things we did was visit Ground Zero; it was our first time back since everything had happened. We just walked around for a while and then just sat there and reflected on what had happened and everything.

Then we started walking to go and have lunch, and I tripped and fell, and hurt my hand but we went on to have lunch, and while we were there my hand started swelling up, so I went to the hospital and it was the same hospital that I was taken to last year. Yes you guessed it, I broke my hand again, the same hand I broke a year earlier. So they casted it, and we went on with our day.

We then went to the Event that night. It was a very nice Event, very Impactful, and the place was packed. My group got to sing the National Anthem. Yes when they introduced us, they told about what had happened to us last year. Then they told about our day leading up to this Event, "They had gone to Ground Zero that morning and that Annie had fallen, and broke the same hand all over again, the same one she broke the year prior."

We stayed for a couple additional days; we had some interviews that were set up prior to our arriving. Then we went back home to Dallas, and I can tell you I was not looking forward to the flight.

Once again when I got home I went and saw my Doctor with my hand and got a new cast, then ten weeks later I finally got it off then I had to start Physical Therapy all over again. I am home again and I am trying to start getting everything back to normal, or as normal as it could be.

A year now has passed by, and I have started once again looking for something to do. I am not one for just sitting around and doing nothing.

I went to Oregon for a couple of weeks to help put on a music camp. I had considered doing something more in the music industry. It was a music camp for children to come and simply study music for the summer. Music lessons would begin at 8 AM and go till about 5 P.M., every night they would have a Jam session so all the students could show off what they learned that day.

Floyd Domino, Chris Booher, Randy Elmore, and Johnny Gimble, http://www.boohermusiccamp.com/instructors.htm , were just some of the artist and teachers that were there. After about a week of this, I knew I did not desire to teach music, I found out that this was not my obsession, I enjoy playing but we are going to leave it at that I am not a teacher.

Consequently on the flight home I am thinking about what I want to do now. I get to talking to the lady sitting next to me, and she is a Travel Agent Instructor, and we talked on the subject of what she does for the majority of the flight, the only thing is I am in the Dallas – Fort Worth area and she was in Phoenix. She told me if I would like to look into it and to even consider it, to just let her know and she would love to give me instructions via the internet, and e-mail.

So I thought about it for awhile, in addition to talking it over with several of my closest friends for their input about what they thought, regarding it. In the mean time she sent me lots of material to study. I like this idea, and I am now thinking I may possibly do this and at the same time I can assist in getting the band to wherever they required being, while they were traveling. I called her and took her up on her proposal, and she then sent me all the material and supplies to get started, she was so sweet and helpful. We did it all via e-mail and the internet; I worked on it every waking second. She told me it would require about a hundred hours to finish.

Well I finished it within just under fifty-eight hours. Now I had to go out and locate an agency to work for. It was great, I found an agency to work under, and I could even work the hours that fit my schedule. I could still be present for the children when it was necessary for me to be with them, and I could even work from my house if I would like to.

Time has gone by, and I currently Love the Travel Industry.
It also goes great with everything else that I'm doing at the present time.

1. Still in my Dance and Music Group

2. Special Feature Planner –find speakers to come in for a local Woman's Group once a month (www. Stonecroft.org)

3. Radio Station – interviewer of special Guest- when artist come into town to promote their New CD – I am the one that interviews them.

4. Piano Lessons – only to a very select view.

5. Choir – Leader

6. Modeling – whenever needed

7. Owner of a Non-Profit agency – I have several people that just look for people around town that we can help. A lot of it comes in at Christmas, but we help them all year long.

8. And if that were not enough I also sell on E-Bay – I am cleaning house, so the next time I move out, I only take what I need.

I have to stay busy, when I am busy doing stuff I don't dwell on everything else that has happened. The Rape, 911, Cancer, Lupus, my Marriage (which is a joke)......

So consequently it is better if I just continue to be active, and to keep putting money into my personal account, so when it comes time for me to leave, I don't have to be concerned about finances. I could even just retire now; I have enough to do me for quite some time. I have already paid off every one of my Credit Cards, as well as my truck.

From this point on, I work for when I am on my own. I know I have to wait till both children are either married, or move out on their own. Which I am looking forward to very much, some days I really don't think it is never going to happen.

Everything at home is presently getting worse. David is getting harder to live with as the days go by; sometimes I question if I will ever be out of this relationship. There are days that I don't believe my children will ever either get married or move out.

Sept 19, 06

I call this the day I finally gave in; well let's back up about a year prior to this point. I was on the Executive Board of Director's of a Group, which was Travel associated. I would go to these meetings once a month. Just about every month this gentleman would talk to me. Not anything further than that, and while we were having our meetings he would constantly sit either alongside me or else in front facing me.

This went on for months, then one day, he asked if he may perhaps come to my agency and talk with me regarding the different companies that he represented, after that we could go have lunch. I said sure, therefore one afternoon he came out to my office and we sat and talked about the company's he represented.

A couple of days went by, and then he called and asked if I needed anything from any of his Clients, and if I would like to go and have lunch with him.

I said: "sure I have something in which I need to talk to you about as well."

Therefore, we met for lunch, and I told him that I had been invited to speak at big conference, at the Convention Center, regarding traveling information and places to go, along with also having a booth so people could pick up information about my Agency and at the same time information on different destinations. I asked him if he would like to assist me with it. He said he would love to lend a hand. This event was in Oct '05'. There were several more Board Meetings, Regular Business Meetings, Lunches and or Dinners that went by.

I remember we went to have lunch one day, and following lunch he walked me to my truck, as he always did, but on this day he walked me to my truck; and we said our Good-Byes and be safe. Then I got inside my truck as he walked to his truck. Then at that moment he looked back over in my direction and had that impression that he had forgotten something, so he walked back over to my truck, I opened up my door and asked:

"If everything was okay, or if there was something wrong?"

He said:

"No I just think I need to kiss you!"

"Let me try to explain."

"When friends meet they often Greet each other by hugging or by kissing."

"I don't want to kiss you out of any Social obligation or because I am worried I will hurt your feelings if I don't, I just think I need to kiss you."

I told him "you know I am married Right?"

He shook his head and said:

"I know, I just thought I needed to give you a Kiss"

We did not kiss. We just said our Good-Byes again. A couple more months went by and several more lunches and dinner meeting went by, and after every Board Meeting that we had, we would meet there early and have a drink, or we would stay late and have a drink, we just enjoyed sitting and talking to each other.

Then shortly thereafter I had a group that I was to take out on a Cruise. Here I was out on this cruise sharing a cabin with two girlfriends, watching couples laugh over dinner, dancing until dawn, and walking hand in hand on the deck.

My life was my many businesses and coexisting at home.

Although it was overpowering at times having a man like William interested in me, I was fearful of disappointing him, once he got to know me better. The life as I now lived was not how I needed to spend the rest of my life. If you don't participate in life, you never get to experience it. The worse that could happen is another man may disappoint me.

William was all I could even think about. I kept thinking about what he had said:

"I just thought I needed to give you a Kiss"

The day after I got back from this cruise I was to be at a travel agent meeting in Dallas at the Renaissance Hotel (Sept 19, 06) and William was present as well. Following this meeting he asked me to join him for a drink at the bar as we have done so many times in the past couple of months.

I said: "sure"

So we sat there and talked for awhile, he was asking me how the trip was with the group and all.

While I was on the cruise I had a pictures made, and he asked if he may possibly have one for him. So I gave him one of the pictures. Then it was time to leave it was getting late. He walked me to my truck. We stood there exchanging the normal pleasantries, then William gave me hug and turned his face to kiss my check as he had respectfully done so many times before. At that time I turned and gave William a kiss and not on the check. I turned my face and softly kissed his lips. You know how they are always saying in the movies that you can tell that you're in Love from the first Kiss? Well now I know it's True.

William looked more quizzical more than surprised.

He said "Goodnight" and started to walk to his truck. He was halfway there, with me still standing in the same spot, watching him go, not knowing his reaction to my kiss, he stopped and looked back at me.

He walked back to me and without saying a word, gently took my face in his hands and kissed me. It was gentle; it was soft and tender and filled with more Love than any Kiss I had ever felt before.

William said:

"It is about time",

Then gave me another short kiss, and said:

"Talk to you tomorrow"

And he turned and left.

Afterwards I had to drive over an hour home, and all that I could even think about was what had just presently happened. I had tears of joy, a smile a mile wide, and my heart filled was filled with something that only love could describe, this was truly something special! Never in my life had I ever felt that way before. I felt special, William brought out feelings that I never knew I had before.

He called the very next day early that morning. Prior to him calling, all I could think about was, did I mess up, the later it got the more:

"I thought that I had messed up, big time."

I really did not think that he would call. Except he did call and wanted to know if we could possibly go and have lunch again. We did and had a fantastic time. A couple of weeks went by of lunches and meetings. Finally, one day he called and asked me to go on an overnight trip with him. He needed to go to Houston for a business meeting for two nights, and if I would like to go.

I thought about it and said:

"Sure, I would love to".

I told David that William was going to pick me up and we were going to go to Houston for two nights, to do some work. At this time David had never met William, therefore they would meet at the time that William was to pick me up to go out of town.

William showed up that morning, William and David met for the first time. David shock William's hand and said: "Have a safe Trip."

Oct 22, 06

William picked me up and we drove to Houston. We talked all the way there about all kinds of stuff, once we got there and got all checked in to our Hotel, we were early for the Event that night, so we went and had a little bite of lunch, and then went back up to our room.

I will tell you I was so nervous, once we got to our room he gave me a Big Hug and Kiss. Then we just sat down on the bed and started talking. Then he turned to me and said something to me that I will by no means never forget. No One had ever asked me anything like that before. He asked: "Can I make Love to you?"

I said "Now?"

I am thinking oh my goodness neither David nor Mike, has ever asked me if they could make love to me, or the fact that it was even in the middle of the day for that matter. The other concern was that No One had ever seen me undressed before.

Married to a buddy, a brother, was extremely emotionally confusing. He was sweet and the kids needed a father figure, but I soon learned why I was wife number two. He was insecure and demanding. What I couldn't give he took. He was half Mike, half housewife with an attitude. Mike had made sex a chore, David made it a non-event. Seventeen years later, David admits he has never seen me nude. William accomplished this our first night away, and taught me to feel good about myself.

Well at this point it is daytime, and William wants to make love to me. Ooh my goodness. Well, he did, and it was Wonderful, and afterwards we just laid there in each other's arms.

Then he looks at me and whispered:

"You just lay here I'm going to get dressed and go get everything situated for the meeting tonight."

"You just get ready and come up whenever you are ready."

"Wow!"

I got up and got ready then went up stairs to the meeting.

After the meeting we went out to dinner, then back to our hotel, we got changed and ready for bed, at this point I was not certain what to imagine. Well he made love to me for a second time. Then he held me in his arms that night as we both sleep together, I have never slept in the arms of someone before, it was absolutely lovely.

Morning came and we made love again. The best part of all of it was that afterwards he would just lay there and hold me in his arms. Well it was now time to get the day started, I went in to take a shower, and I have always taken a shower with the lights off because I do not desire to observe myself any more than I have to.

Plus I was in the shower when the first plane hit during 911, every once in awhile I will hear some noise and the memories of that day come back. So ever since then, I have taken showers in the dark using just the light from the other room. Plus I have so many scars, physical and emotional, that I just don't like looking at myself, and I have gained so much weight since then that I just really don't want to see myself in the mirror.

At that moment while in the shower, William has stuck his head in and asked if he may possibly join me? I remember screaming from surprise because it frightened me so much. My first thought was 911, and after that my next thought was No

One has ever seen me undressed, nor have I ever taken a shower with somebody else. No one has even ever asked if they could take a shower with me.

We did take a shower together, however at first William just stood there and held me till I got over the shock of the scare. It was a Wonderful Shower.

The morning after, I showered for the first time with a man. It's my favorite way to start a day. We then got dressed and ready for the day. The rest of the day all I could think about was that No one had ever seen me undressed, and that whenever he dropped me off at home, that I would most likely never hear from him again.

That I would only see him at meetings and that is all we would have together. Boy was I wrong; he called me that night along with the next day. He told me that he had a Wonderful time. William then even gave me some additional dates that he was going to have to be out of town and would love it if I could join him.

"Wow He likes me!"

Weeks went by and more and more trips, Houston, Austin, San Antonio, New Orleans...... then came Dec and I had to go to Mexico with my band group, to do a performance there. William could not come on this trip for some reason, and it was on this trip I realized not only that I missed him very much, but that I also Loved him Very Much.

Right before I went on this trip I had a Doctor appointment, to have some blood work done. The Doctor called me the next day and told me that my Lupus was in complete remission.

Wow I could not think of anyone else that I would have rather been with when I found out. William put his arms around me and just held me, and was telling me how proud he was. Then we got dressed up and went out and had a celebration dinner.

The next day I left for Mexico for a week, and while on this trip I fell and broke my hand again. (yes the same one that I broke during 911). After I left the hospital the only thing I wanted to do was to talk with William, well I was able to get a hold of him on my cell phone and talk to him.

He said:

"Baby it will be okay"

"We will work around it."

"Don't worry about it. I am going to be here for you,"

And he was. He was so helpful when we were together.

Unlike whenever I was at home with David he would just say:

"oh well"

There were times that I would be in need, of help to put something on or to open something, but No help.

He would just say:

"What if I was not here?"

So from then on I would make sure that whatever I was going to wear or do that I would not have to ask for his help.

It is now Jan '07' and I'm still in a cast, I have to take a group out, and William is having to take a group out as well. So we are not together but we talked several times a day. I missed him very much, and I don't think that I have ever missed anybody as much as I missed him on this trip.

After we got home, we got together and spent some time together. This was the first time that he bought me a piece of jewelry. It is the most beautiful piece ever; it is a Heart pendant with a Gaspeite Stone in the middle. It is just spectacular looking. Oh my goodness I cannot believe he has bought this for me, it is so beautiful.

Then in February, I had to go to Tennessee, with my performance group, with another singing group that I am a part of. While I was there all I could think about is when I get home William is going to be there to pick me up at the airport, and we are going to San Antonio for a couple of days, and it was going to fall over Valentine's Day. I was so looking forward to this so very much. I have never really ever liked Valentine's Day before, because as I told you David and I were never really in Love so we never really did the whole Valentine – Heart Sweet stuff thing, or the whole Christmas thing for that matter.

So therefore I was very much looking forward to Valentine's Day this year. I had bought three boxes of rose petals and on the morning of Valentines, while William was in the bathroom I threw them all over the room, and in the bed and everywhere. You should have seen his face when he came out.

William gave me a piece of him for Valentine's Day. He gave me a locket that he looked all over town for, and in this locket he put a piece of his hair, because I am always playing with his hair, and a Star of David. That way I would always have a piece of him with me at all times. I had the locket put on my charm bracelet. From this point on, if he did not have a meeting out of town some where we would stay overnight in a local hotel. No it wasn't about sex many nights it was just about sleeping in each other's arms, I generally don't sleep well when I am at home.

It is now May and we went out on our first real none working trip. We went out on a short cruise; it was our first real trip together. We had a Blast, everyone thought that we were on our Honeymoon; William would tell them:

"Yes we are on our Pre-Honeymoon".

They would all say that they could see how much we were in Love with one another. On one of our stops was in was Cozumel; while we were there William had one thing he was looking for, prior to the cruise I had lost my thumb ring, and he wanted to replace it. We looked in every single jewelry store there in Cozumel. William found several that we liked, then he found it the ring that would be my new thumb ring, he put it on and told me it was only temporary.

I may never find the right words to express how William has made me feel... he has brought out so many feelings. Even the feeling of that I am a Woman; he even treats me like a woman.

Then June came and we went out on our next trip, we went out on the Train. We boarded the train in Las Vegas, and went up Salt Lake City, Yellowstone, Grand Tetons, and Jackson Hole. We had yet another Wonderful time. Neither of us had ever been to any of these places so it was great to see them together.

This was another Wonderful and memorable Trip. During the day we went out and saw the city that we were in. At night the train would travel to the next stop. Well we both slept in a Twin size bed while the train was Traveling; William would hold me all night so that I would not fall out of the bed.

Then July came and I got really sick. I met William for lunch one day and was telling him that my chest was hurting very bad, not like a heart attack or anything like that; it was just right in the middle of my chest. So then while on my way home I called and made a Doctor appointment. It was late in the day on July 3, and the next appointment time I could get was the morning of July 5. So William said:

"I will come and take you to the Doctor"

"So just plan on it"

"I will be there in the morning to pick you up to take you to the Doctor"

So on the 4th of July I just went to a friend's house for a 4th of July Party. And really did not do much, and that is when my friend's knew something was wrong. Because I didn't go swimming or anything, I just sat and watched them.

Then the next day William came to take me to the Doctor. They took Cat-Scans, and some other test. That evening, shortly after I got home, the Dr called and told me to go to the hospital right then; I was talking to William on the other line when the Doctor called. So once I was finished talking with the Doctor I went back over to tell William what the Doctor said, along with that he wanted me to go straight to the hospital and that he would call the hospital and have them waiting on me to for when I got there. He said that I had a pretty good size blood clot in my liver, lungs and in my kidney's.

David was out in the garage working on his truck, I went out and told him that the Doctor had called and for me to go to the Emergency Room, and that he was calling the hospital ahead, to have some specialist there waiting for me. Mean while I still had William on the phone and he could hear everything that was going on. He overheard David say well let me get done working on the truck here, and then we can go.

I could hear William yelling:

"NO"

"You tell him you have to go NOW."

This was the first time that William really understood what I was talking about, that there really was not any love here.

William was there with me every day. He would massage and put lotion on my back and feet every day. He was there with me everyday most of all day; David would just come and go. Every time I would have some test done William was there plus he was always waiting for me once I came out of the testing. Even when I got out of the hospital he came over to the house to visit and to keep me company.

I am getting better, and for awhile we did not go out of town or go anywhere. William would just come to the house to be with me. We just kind of took it easy for awhile. We were working on getting me better because I had a huge dance cruise coming up in September, which I in reality needed to be on. William had to go out of town somewhere during this cruise so he was unable to go with me.

So I found a friend from within the dance group to be my roommate. This cruise would also fall over the Anniversary of 911. I have currently gotten to the point that I do not like being at home during this time frame; I would like to be away somewhere. I explained to the lady staying in the room with me about 911. She was very supportive, that night at Dinner the ship crew did a little Anniversary song in Honor of 911, it was done very well.

The day that William and I celebrate our Anniversary is September 19; I call this the day that I gave in. Well the plans were, I was going to go on the cruise, come home and the very next day we were to go to Florida for a concert and TV interview that I was doing there with my group. On my way home from the cruise, I tried calling him several times and never got a hold of him. I was getting very worried.

Finally after a couple of hours we connected, and he was in the hospital, William remained in the hospital most of a week. It wasn't anything major just a sensitive area that had to heal before he was released.

Therefore, William was not going to be able to go to Florida, and by this point I actually did not desire to go anymore, it was our Anniversary and I had gotten us a room at a hotel away from the rest of the group and on the beach.

So now the next thing we had to look forward to was going to go on a cruise at the end of October, so we just started getting everything ready for that. As the day got closer, I got more and more excited, we were going to be away just the two of us, no work, no one that we have to watch out for or anything like that.

It is the day and we met at the airport, and oh my goodness people that we both knew were there and if that was not bad enough they were even on the same flight with us to Miami, Florida. They were going somewhere else but it was very frustrating.

We get to Miami, Florida and caught the shuttle over to the ship. This was the best cruise that we have been on it was a seven day cruise, and we had an amazingly, wonderful time. We did all kinds of excursions together, William loves to be as active as me, and I really love that about him. He does not like to just sitting still, however we do both know at what time to just sit and enjoy one another. It was also on this trip that William bought me another ring, this ring was a very special ring, and it replaced my existing wedding ring. He said he it was a ring for me to wear so that I would know how much he loved me and that I could wear it till the day that he could replace it with a Wedding Ring on our Wedding Day.

Well we are currently back home, and still enjoying one another. Then within a month or so after we were home I found out that I was pregnant. William and I were out of town for just an overnight away, and that is when I told him that I thought that I might be pregnant, that I was really late. William assured me that everything was going to be okay! That we would work through it.

So I called and made an appointment to go in and see the Doctor. The only thing bad concerning all of this is, a couple of years ago my Doctor told me not to get pregnant again. That it was not good for my health, and there was a strong probability that it could even cause death, so you see this was not good news at all.

Before we could talk more about what we were going to do, one night I was laying in bed and did not feel well at all. William was out of town, so I couldn't call him and everybody else was away as well. So I drove myself to the hospital, where later I had a miscarriage.

Once William got back in town he came immediately over to where I was and he just held me.

WOW GOOD NEWS

My daughter's boy friend has asked me if he may ask my daughter to marry him~! My first reaction was No way! I did not know him that well and was not sure if I liked him yet or not, but I said yes, after all it is her decision. Then I was hit with rethinking my feelings about her marriage. Is this guy a Mike or a David? Will this man cause my daughter to walk the steps of my life? I then realized that this is my daughter who I helped learn as she grew. She is wise and insightful, and she chooses her friends well. This guy had to be more William than a Mike or David. Then there was the fact that her happiness will bring me closer to mine.

Well the children have picked a date and have started planning everything. I think that was the hardest part for them, because he is in the military and he is overseas, so the wedding as of right now is planned for March 26, 2010. They have picked their colors, which are going to be green and white; they have even started getting all the other details in order. They have even started getting a guest list together.

At this moment my soul purpose is to start getting all my finances in order, to make sure they are all right where they need to be. I am now working even harder at getting everything prearranged so I will have everything where I need it to be when the time gets here.

I know it is going to be two years before the children get married, but with that it gives me time to get everything else arranged. Since I don't want them to get married one day, move out the next, and then I move out the next. I will wait for a little while afterwards before I do move out. I don't ever want the children to think that I was waiting on them before I did anything. They do not even have a clue that I am even thinking of moving out. They are under the impression that everything at home is great. They do not need to know any different right now.

David or Mike

Lately David is getting to be more and more a lot like Mike. Just the other day I was trying to fix something for the children, I had told the children that I would fix them breakfast in the morning. Oh No David did not think that I could do it. I was going to fix pancakes, big deal, but oh no he had to take the measuring cup away from me. He was going to do it, because I would screw it up. So I just went ahead and let him do it, well then he wanted to put stuff in the batter that I can't eat. When I pointed it out he swung the glass measuring cup and hit me in the nose and gave me a black eye.

After all these years my family has not changed a great deal. They still don't come to my house. They are jealous of what I have achieved plus what I have. If my Mom comes out to my house just once in six months, that would be really a lot for her. In addition, I would be stunned. I don't believe she likes David, except she won't say so. Then if I don't go to her house at least once a week I am black balled along with being talked about. My Mom only lives about twenty minutes max away from me. Numerous times I would call her and invite her to come out so we could perhaps go to eat or else go shopping. Nope, I have to go to her place, and after that we could set out from there.

One of my brothers as well as sisters lives about two hours away. My Mom goes to their house at least twice a month, and she has to go right passed my house. I have asked her on her way there or else on her way home to stop by. Well you know the response to that one.

Of the nine children who are still alive four of my brothers and sisters, have never been to my house. They won't even know how to find my house.

Christmas '07'

We were suppose to of have Christmas at my house, but a couple of days prior to Christmas every one decided not to come that they would just hang about at home. The day prior to Christmas my Mom called me to let me know the intention of what was going to take place;

We are all going to have Christmas at her house.

It is now Christmas time and William has just given me a New Puppy for Christmas. I had a dog previously, but he ran away while we were away on a trip. The new puppy is so cute; this will be my first ever big dog. We have named the dog Love. I know I have gotten grief from everybody about the dog's name, but he (Love) loves his name. Whenever I say "Love" he just comes running. He is not having any difficulty with his name, and that is all that matters.

I just looked up Loves Birth date, Oh my goodness Loves birth date is the same identical date just a year later that William made Love to me for the first time. Loves birth date is Oct. 22, 2007

William and I have been talking about getting a place of our own, an apartment in which we could meet, as an alternative to meeting in the parks, restaurant or a hotel here or there, we were always renting a hotel for a day at least twice a week. Just so that we could have a place to hang out together.

"Doing the math"

As William likes to say, it was cheaper. Than going to a hotel all the time. Now we could just get together at our place. We started looking, and I told him that I also had a storage unit full of furnishings, that were left over from my previous move that I never moved to the house. So we would have a good start.

We found the ideal place, put down a deposit. Then I went to the storage space to kind of take an inventory of what was in there. Then I went shopping and start getting things that I knew we were going to need when we moved in. We were to move in mid Jan after we got back from another trip that we previously had planned.

Jan 08

William and I went to Vegas for a week. We had a magnificent time. I can sincerely say no matter where we go or what we do we have a grand time. William and I went to one of the shows that I had gone to previously, and I enjoyed it so greatly that I wanted to experience it with William. We also went to other shows while we were there. We walked around and visited some of the other resorts. We stayed at the New York New York. After my encounter with New York and 911 we worried about how I would do there but it all turned out just fine.

William and I moved into our New apartment.

The day is here and we are going to meet at the storage space and move stuff into the apartment. Since it was a one bedroom and we both had trucks, it only took us three loads to get it all there. We did it all together, got everything in the apartment then started getting it all unpacked and put away. Once that was all completed we went and bought some groceries. Then we spent the first night at our place. I had not ever gone grocery shopping with David before. He would never go with me whenever I would ask him to go. As a matter of fact I cannot think of a single thing that

David and I, that we have done together, we always did things within a group of friends. I would recommend things to do, and he never wanted to.

Well William and I have had our apartment for over a year now, and it is great! We get together there just about every day of the week, even if it is for just a couple of hours at a time. Just to have lunch, or to just sit around and talk, we just take pleasure in being in each other's company.

We have even had several overnights there as well, even when we go out of town we try and have our last night out at the apartment, if someone were to walk into the apartment, they would think that we have been there for awhile, we have already gotten just about everything we need. We have really enjoyed decorating the place together.

Holding Hands

Sometimes the smallest things, too many the most common gestures, are the most difficult to comprehend. As an infant either Momma or Papa took my hand to teach me to walk. My brothers Ryan and Tyler took my hand to cross the street or to visit neighbors. I held hands with classmates when traveling from the class to the playground, from the lunch room to the gym. I hold hands with dance partners and sometimes when I sing a duet.

Holding hands is support, direction, a sense of being joined, security, but on the first day I walked with William and he reached out and took my hand, holding hands took on a meaning I had never experienced before. The support was a sense of:

"I am here with you to help you find your way."

The direction was:

"Here we are and we are going together".

The sense of security was something I had never knowingly experienced before.

His hand in mine, are fingers entwined like an arm around my shoulders. It kept harm, it made me feel safe. It calmed me and reduced the stress throughout my body. No word necessary, just a sense of well being. Forty years of chaos brought to a screaming halt by five fingers and a hand.

February

Can you believe that it is Feb. again already? This year we spent Valentine's Day in Houston, it was great we had a Wonderful time. Then we went to Oklahoma City for me to do a photo shoot, along with going to a late Valentines Dinner with some friends.

It is great having the apartment, because I love to cook and we have been able to cook meals together. We have dinner in our own place several times. We just go to the store and get only what we need for that meal. Since we are not there all the time we don't really buy a lot so that it can just sit around and waste.

Talking with William

One of the hardest parts of my relationship with William is being open and honest. I always had to hide everything from everyone and old habits die slow. William and I are starting to have problems, he needs an open relationship and I haven't learned to open up yet. The yellow brick road to happiness has a few ruffles and flourishes, a bolder of two and a learning curve. I know I Love William and I know William truly Loves me, I am still walking the road to that reality. We have started over coming this and we both talk to one another about everything. We both know that it is going to be hard, for me because for so many years I have not been able to speak my mind, if I were to open my mouth and talk I would get either knocked around, or I would get "you don't know what you are talking about talk."

We work together more, business works, we are a great team, two peas in a pod and learning everything else from each other. We have taken groups out together and what I used to do wonderfully by myself has turned into magic, with his old world charm and sophistication. With my imagination and William's, what each misses the other gets. Even friends are starting to notice the difference in me. I have always shown a happy face, now it's no longer just an image, it's real.

Then during the month of February and March I stayed at the apartment just so I could get away and think about everything that was going on.

William came over during the day. At night I would just sit and relax and think about what was going on and what I was going to do. He had to go out of town for awhile during this time, on a business trip and when he was due home I picked him up at the airport, and he was able to stay overnight at our place before he went home.

Hotel Shooting

Just because Mike is behind me, and David is soon to follow don't think live has gotten dull. There is lots of traveling in my other career in the Travel Industry.

Doing Sales Calls, a night here and a day there. Most of the excitement of my nights is shared with William. Others come from things like the morning when Williams went out to get something, and there was a shooting in the room next door to mine.

Living through Mike's trigger happen days, and 9-11 causes moments like this to be even more traumatic. Apparently the hotel was not even aware of what occurred, the Police came and went and everything was cleaned up that fast.

When I related what had happened to the woman at the front desk and we got into my past experiences and this book I am writing. She asked for a copy to share with a friend who is living through a similar tragedy. She hoped that her friend might learn from my life and be better equipped to survive.

Traveling with my Group

This coming March we are going to Florida for a week, my group is going to be performing there, and William has not yet gotten to see me on stage. I am very nervous about this, but I know it will be good for the both of us, even for William to get to see me perform on stage, and at the same time William will get to meet the rest of the group.

Then in April I have to go to New York City to help out at The Juilliard School for a dance class, that is where I went to school for my music, during my High School Years, and they have asked me and a couple of others to come and teach some classes. I told them it would be an Honor to come and teach. William is going to join me there for about a week.

Talking with David

David and I don't hardly talk anymore, it is hard for me to even look him in the eye and talk to him, the last time we had a real talk was right after I got out of the hospital, and we were talking about our relationship, and how we felt about each other, we talked about it for quite some time and we agreed that we were more like brother and sister, instead of husband and wife. What makes this even harder is that none of our friends, or family even know anything about it, they all think that we are just a Happily Married Couple!

David and I went out to eat the other day, just David and I, we sat there for two hours and never said a word to one another. I saw some friends there and went over and talked with them for a minute. They invited us to join them, but it was best at this point not to join them.

Every week it is the same old thing, I go to choir practice on Wednesday and Sunday Nights, Saturday Night we have a group of friends that we go to Dinner with, then we have to go to a movie, Church on Sunday Morning, with the same group of friends, we go to one of our houses and have lunch, every week it is at a different friends house. With this same group of friends every year we all go on a trip together somewhere, even if it is just for overnight, David and I always have to go behind their back and talk to the hotel and tell them we need two beds please. Therefore we never invite our friends into our room. We always meet in the lobby or in another friend's room.

My heart just breaks for the reason that now all I can reflect on is about how much I desire to be with William. If I could leave this marriage tomorrow I would. I recognize I'm a full-grown woman, I have plenty of funds to accomplish whatsoever I would like to achieve. At the present time cannot do that to my children, which at this point in time they are nineteen and twenty. Of course they are extremely close to being on the course of being away from home and on their own. It is simply a matter of time; I can now see the light at the other end. This is making it a little easier.

Every night all David talk's about is how I do everything wrong, in regards to everything, cooking, cleaning, my business's, along with that I couldn't achieve no matter what without him around to hold me up.

To him I don't even dress right; he is forever asking me:

"Why did you get that?" Or

"You are going to wear that?"

Subsequently I have other people telling me how greatly they like whatever it is that I am wearing. As a result every now and then I don't know what to believe. Am I dressing nice or else just strange and weird?

However if I like the outfit I just continue wearing it, I in actuality don't really worry about it! In addition William is at all times telling me that I dress very nice.

William has been a breath of fresh air. He comes from an upscale lifestyle where he knows and appreciates clothes. He dresses very well and understands woman's fashions. I never had a man ever go shopping with me but William not only asks to go, he also picks out outfits. He has changed my thinking about styles and colors, as a lot of my thinking goes back to my old size Twenty-six.

He even knew my sizes as they started to drop before I realized the difference. His new direction is getting me into light colored and white pants and shirts. Now that I have more attractive legs my skirts have gotten shorter. He has even effected my choice of lingerie, bra's used to be strictly utilitarian just something to cover and hold up my big boobs.

Now they are silky and lacey. Panties were cotton covers, now they are silks and satin, lace and a little peek-a-boo. Before I was afraid to be seen, now I'm getting to like the body I see. William has even bought me to a certain extent a reasonably amount of my fresh new outfits. Not only does he know what size I wear, he knows what I like.

As far as losing the weight, I just told myself it had to be done. So I started eating less, a little at a time. Nothing major, just small amounts. As well as I gave up soft drinks. That is all I did. No fancy Diet program or anything, just cut my meals down and ate less.

Surgery

After numerous surgeries; repairing body damage at the hands of Mike, Cancer, breast reduction, esophagus replacement, removing a blood clot, repairing broken legs and arms, you would think that the last thing I would entertain is the idea of another surgery. Well, my Hematology and Oncology (blood Dr) Doctor decided that if I had this special surgery, one affecting my hormones, that it would help correct other blood related problems in my body. Namely minimize if not eliminate the threat of blood clots. So here I go again. This one was a partial hysterectomy, day surgery.

You know how I never do things the easy way. Not to disappoint anyone, the surgery went perfect accept for some reason the internal stitches which should have been gone in a week, took two months. The Doctor could only assume that with all the changes in medication in my body, mainly being taken off all my meds for the first time in 20 years, that the immune system was taking longer to heal itself, it hadn't had to do it without help for a long time.

Now the happy ending to this segment of the story. After all these years of health problems, three - four different medications a day, weekly visits to one Doctor or another, this is where I am. I now take zero medication, all my former ailments are in remission or gone, and the Doctor's say my next visit is not in a week or a month, but now yearly. All the spots on the paper are the tears of joy that I unashamedly shed.

Grape Stomp

It's June and I just realized that William has a Birthday not to far down the road. It's funny in two years I have gone from no partner, with no involvement, to what can we do next.

"We" what a Wonderful word.

I sat down at the computer and started a trek across Texas. Well not really across Texas, I just started from home and spread the map out further and further. Somewhere around Austin all those Wineries started to pop up. He likes wine, and he has mentioned an attempt to grow his own. He has even said:

"Once I retire I want to move to Northern California and buy a Wine Vineyard," "nothing big just enough grapes to ensure that the Wine Cellar is never empty."

Well just outside of New Braunfels there is this place called:

"Comal Creek Vineyards" that offers an Event called:

"Order of the Purple Foot"

It's a Grape Stomp with a TWIST. Designed "for adult couples only", this event assigns one person to do the "stomping" and the other to do the "collecting".

The couple producing the most juice in the allotted time wins. One prize will go to the overall winner and inclusion of their names on a permanent plaque displayed proudly in the Tasting Room.

On July 29, 2008 we drove to the Winery. There were about a hundred-twenty other wine-o's there, the set up was very cute. Twenty wooden barrels, hoses and plastic bottles for gathering the juice, Twenty pairs of contestants per round competing, to see who could stomp the most juice out of eight pounds of grapes. I don't know if it was the competition, or the new friends that we made that were more fun.

Two couples were from Houston who came together, another couple was from Lake Charles LA, William and me. We all hit it off right from the start, and we all shared our cameras so that we could have pictures, of our experience. There was a lovely gift shop to taste test wines, and all the related gifts and gadgets for Wine.

The competition started with twenty teams of two manning the wooden barrel in which the grapes were thrown. One of us, me, because I have the larger feet to stomp the grapes, the other to gather the drippings.

Ten minutes to stomp, drip, and gather the juice.

Purple feet, hands and clothes. Lots of laughs, cheering, and advice from the on lookers who did not know anymore about what to do then we did. In the end we wound up Third out of our group of Twenty, and something like ninth or tenth out of all sixty couples.

Then there was lunch, lots more wine to taste and to enjoy. Great conversation, we then all went and made Purple foot prints on the back of our T-Shirts that we got at the Event, we made the foot prints with the grape juice that we had collected from the stomp. But most important, William had a different Birthday which he Loved, and I got to be with my guy, doing something together.

Trip to Mexico

In August 2008 as part of one of my many businesses it was necessary to introduce Travel Agents to one of the Resorts which I represented. I had been on FAMS, "Familiarization Trips" many times, but as a guest. William being in another side of the Travel Industry had escorted many such trips, and I asked him to help me plan, suggest people to ask, and come along to help the trip be a success.

"Duh! Yes" and for us to have time together.

All seventeen of us arrived in drips and drabs on the same day. The Hotel had arranged for shuttles for each of the arrivals to be taken to the hotel. The Group came from all around the country. A couple of them where travel agents who worked for me. The whole idea of this trip was for the Agents to become familiar with the Resort, fall in love with it, and send lots of clients here.

I also had an underlining reason for some of the Guests. I wanted some of my friends to meet Williams. Most important were Cory and John, two of my closest friends. They have a great relationship and are fun people and I both wanted and needed their approval. We had five days of sightseeing, visiting some other hotels, trying out all of the restaurants, lounging, and drinking by the pool, the guys checking out all the topless sun bathers, and lots of laughs.

In the end, William felt it was necessary to be up front and sat down with John and told him about us. John was sort of aware and when we spoke to Cory she said:

"I have never seen my friend Annie, happier than I am seeing her right now, and you know what, that is all that matters to me, that is all that is really important."

David

After 17 years of friendship, and his help caring for the children and the house, what is making David expendable. I have spoken of his lack of interest in the things I do and his participation. David is also the second coming of Mike. Well in all fairness not really, he is unreasonable and abusive, both verbally and physically, but where Mike threw me through windows, stabbed me with a knife and shot me, just for fun, David is more a show of strength. Like squeeze a leg or choke a throat or leave a mark to remind me he is the stronger one. If I rated some of the things he does I wouldn't like it but I could in a moment of weakness take some responsibility, but no one's imagination can stretch that far.

A couple of day ago my Dad came to visit, and since he came and I did not let David know that he was coming, it angered David very much. Once my Dad was gone he tried to strangle me because of it. By week's end I needed all new make up to replace the heavy coverage that was necessary to keep the world from noticing the bruises. This was followed by another session because I cooked dinner and he believes he is the better cook, so I am not supposed to cook anything.

Relationships, as I have learned with Williams are joint ventures, working together, and not some competition where someone has to win, or more importantly where someone has to lose.

Closing

So here I am. David has moved out and hopefully will move on. My Daughter when she marries will be busy traveling around the world. I have William, I believe. We are still developing a wonderful relationship, but it is two years in the making, and when I walk down that road, that aisle again, I will know that this is truly until do us part.

On New Year's Eve William wrote me the following:

On this evening, on the dawning of a new year.

A year that marks the beginning of our two lives forever after.

On this your first New Years Eve out on the town.

Sharing with the first man who will share each day with you forever.

And although I can only love you for the rest of my life.

I will fill your days with enough love that you will love me for the rest of your life.

It was very hard getting here, but it is a wonderful place to be.

Modeling Events:

The cycle of life being ever changing, I have gotten back into my first love, my modeling career. The way this came about is a Wonderful friend of mine John called, who used to be my agent, until I got out of modeling, because of all the scars and everything else. John would have me modeling on behalf of different commercials, in addition to article ads. John was looking at getting back into the industry, and he wanted to get re-establish with me. So the next step was he scheduled me a photo shoot.

Some Additional Funny Stories

Airline Trips:

Corpus Christi

I was departing to Corpus Christi for the weekend. The whole thing was going great. Got to the airport and before long, it was time to begin boarding the Flight. It was open seating so you had to get there before departure time to wait in line. I was one of the ones near the beginning.

We started the process of boarding the airplane; I got a seat close up to the front and by the window. After that a gentleman sat in the aisle sit, and then he started holding his stomach to saying:

"I believe I am going to get sick; it must have been something that I ate for Dinner last night."

After a short while of this he leans over in my direction and says:

"I am not under the weather however I'm going to act as if I am, therefore maybe we be able to maintain this seat empty."

I told him: "go right ahead."

"I would Love for the seat to be empty with the intention of not being stuffed in here at this time."

St. Louis

Now I'm at the airport getting prepared to go to St. Louis. And the gate representative has just walked thru and announced that, they are going to have a weighing machine at the gate, and it is meant for each person to get on with their carry-ons to be weight so they could possibly level out the weight. That the luggage compartment was overweight, therefore they were going to have to reshuffle the passengers in the effort to work it out. And three passengers did not make that departure that day due to heaviness of their belongings and everything.

Kansas Trip:

Well at the present time I am departing on my way to Kansas to visit a friend of mine. We loaded the flight, and the flight attendant completed all the announcements they constantly make, and said:

"As in a little while as soon as we obtain to cruising altitude I will be through to provide beverages."

This was going to be an extremely short flight like barely an hour to an hour and half. Well a little while later I overheard a number of the other passengers discussing something, so I started listening.

The flight attendant had FALLEN SOUND ASLEEP in her jump seat. We never did obtain a drink that day. At that time the pilot came on and told everybody to get prepared for landing and that the flight attendant would be through the cabin to collect any trash that we might have. Every looked at one another and asked what flight attendant? And what trash we never got a drink or anything to create trash? In addition to that she never moved. I wish I could have had a camera on behalf of everybody present for when we landed the expression on her face was beyond priceless.

Once we landed I called a friend of mine back home that does the teaching and trains the flight attendants in the DFW area, and told her of what happened. She was very angry. Then she said something extremely interesting, you know that is a High-Jacker's Dream. Or what if somebody would have had a Heart Attack?

April Fool's Day

I remember one April Fool's Day – I was out of town with my group and we were at the hotel having a meeting in the conference room. At first I did not realize that it was April Fool's Day. Once I found out it was all over, the only problem was, I was out of town in a hotel and had not planned anything. Then I overheard one of the other guy's asking about where the coffee was, I thought for a minute and then I said hold up I will get it for you.

Plan went in to action, the coffee – I went in to the kitchen and ask the staff about some coffee. But told them it could not be regular ordinary coffee. We had to Dr it up a little after all it was April Fool's Day. So we took a bunch of different flavored soda's along with some coffee, mixed it all up then ran it through that coffee pot so that it would be nice and hot for them, after all you can't serve them cold coffee.

One of the older gentlemen of the group saw me carrying the coffee pot and asked for some, I really did not want to get him, so I told him really sweet like;

"You really don't want any of this coffee!"

"You need to wait on the other pot."

He did not take the hint and followed me to my first victim; I gave one of the guy's a coffee cup and poured him some coffee, then went to the next, so on, and so on. They just put their creamers and sugar in it and then one of them took a drink, and then he looked at me and said:

"WHAT kind of coffee is this?"
I said real nice like once again:
"Is there something wrong with it?"
Then one of them said:
"There is something wrong with this coffee"
And then one of them saw me smirk. He said:
"There is something wrong with this coffee look at her!"
I just looked at all of them and said: "April Fool's ~!~!"

Love Letters and Text messages to Annie from William

Christmas without
Hear the soft sound of falling snowflakes,
Through the town a sleigh glides down the road,
Colored lights are twinkling around windows
Neighbors hurrying home with their shopping loads.
In a window on the second floor,
With a view clear down the street,
William's a lonely figure searching,
Waiting for their eyes to meet.
A car goes by and then another,
A taxi slows but never stops,
And the gift of love that begs delivery,
Will it be left in the shop?
So we each stand waiting in our windows,
With hope, separated by our front doors,
Knowing that the gift we want for Christmas,
Is each others' PRESENCE and nothing more.

Loving you
I wish I had the years back,
To be 40 again, but you still 39,
More years in which to Love you,
To be loved by you.
But since those can be but wishes
I promise you this reality,
I will take the best care of me,
To make this body ready
To fill your heart with Love,
For as much time as possible
To fill your body with endless
Moments of passion and ecstasy
Because I do Love You
Where would my life be without Annie?
Would my heart beat as strong?
This smile, would it be on my face,
When I sleep at night, would I rest?
And would I care as much if tomorrow came.

I love Paris in the Springtime.
I love standing on a Street corner in Brooklyn in the Summer.
I love New England and its Fall Foliage.
I love Banff all covered with snow.
I am going to spend the rest of my life loving you.

I sit here suspended in mid air,
As if time is standing still,
Life is not an up, nor am I down,
Heavy is my burden of waiting.
Martin Luther King had a dream,
I have the reality that is you,
A bullet kept him from realizing his,
I live 50 miles away from mine.
Help me find the way to you,
Lead me through the discovery of Annie,
Let me make your world what you deserve,
I want each of our lives to be together.

As a little girl you had a path,
You'd grow and be this Lady,
The child a Mother would become,
A women and a Lover.
And now some pages have come true,
Others are still waiting,
You need to walk at least half the way,
If you want life to have full meaning.
A man waits down the road,
To fill your life and heart,
He can't do it all alone,
You'll have to share a part.
How much will you let me teach you?
How much must I learn,
I love standing there beside you,
When not there I just yearn,
The shine that burns in those brown eyes,
That smile which lifts my heart,
Such warmth when enfolded in your arms,
Feeling secure even when apart,
This is my love with you.

If I were to work out 8 hours each day for 30 years,
I would not have the strength which your love gives me.
On in death would I be calm,
relaxed and have the sense of peace you bring into my life,
My vision and insight are magnified through the things which
you have experienced,
I am becoming all the Man I hoped to achieve because of your
Love,
I once had a fantasy that two people could share in making love
and the passion would be equally experienced.
Annie, you make that fantasy a reality.
I do Love You.

Slowly the sun's rays reach over the horizon,
Like finger tips
It brings beauty to the morning
Embracing me with warmth like being snuggled in your arms
Waves wash the shore, refreshing and cleansing the land
Like sharing a shower with you
While your hands caress my body
Birds flutter through trees
Bunnies nibble on Flowers
Sleepy Reeds rise up to meet the sun.
Like your kisses which awake me,
The sweet essence of your body,
And the arousal you stimulate
With your Finger Tips
All things Natural and Beautiful,
The expressions of Love which you
Bring into my Life each morning.

As we lay here side by side I feel the softness and the strength of your body.

I am surrounded by the need to bring you joy.

Moving from being lost in your eyes to placing my lips on yours.

Feeling their warmth and tenderness, sensing you passion.

Stroking those lips with my tongue, gently nibbling.

Fluttering kisses across your eyes, over the edge of your check, sliding down your neck.

My mouth moves not for words, but to enclose an ear.

To trace the curve of that sea shell with the tip of my tongue,

I hear a sigh, "oh yes".

I feel your breast against my chest like two down pillows, reaching to cup one in my hand.

Running my lips around each mound, taking you into my mouth, I feel them filling.

Exploding from each center a now rigged nipple pointing for attention. Moistened by my lips, encircled, suckled, and aroused.

I slide across the comforter of the bed and down your side, stopping at the crescent of your bellybutton.

Probing it's depth, feeling muscles ripple in response.

And now that scent I sensed while traveling from your neck and across your chest, and down your belly.

It is the pure sweetness of you.

It is a mixture of love and passion and made up of fluids of your being.

A hillock, a down covered rise.

Peeking through and into the entrance of the valley.

A single Rosebud pushed to the surface.

Using gentle fingers to move the hillsides of the valley.

I take this flower between two soft fingers and caress it.

I take it in to my lips and shower it with kisses,

I hungrily take it in my mouth and rake it with my teeth.

My ears are pounded with your "oh yeses" and sighs of joy.

My hands encircling your buttocks and being slapped by your rapid rising and falling against them.

I bury my face in the valley, trying to reach your depth.

My tongue stoking the furthest reaches of that canal, I take the lips which form the hillsides and devour them.

While again stroking that rosebud of your passion.

Louder become your exclamations of sexual joy.

Stronger are the leapings of your body.

Then there is a straining and rigidity of muscles in the throws of Orgasm.

I take you in my arms and gently let the feelings slowly ebb and flow, sharing in your enjoyment of the feelings through every fiber of your body. Waiting for the feeling to subside, but never totally leave, never totally leaving for one moment for the rest of our life.

A light to turn on and feel its glow by just saying my Name, and I Love You

Sometimes I think about
the first time I realized that I love you...
It was as if my eyes
took a picture at that moment
and stored it in my heart.
Sometimes I think about
how much my life has changed
because of you.
I think about you
and your happiness...
about us
and about our life together...
and I realize that you are
as much a part of me now
as the air I breathe
and the Dreams I nurture.
But from time to time,
I still like to remember
the first time
I looked into your eyes
and saw my future there.

It isn't easy
being so in love with you
and not being able to see you
every day. There are times
when I'd give anything
just to be able
to gaze into your eyes
or hold you in my arms,
even for a few minutes.
I always feel incomplete,
like a part of me is missing,
when we're not together.
I know that, right now,
this is how things have to be,
but that doesn't make it
any easier to bear.
Every day without you
just reminds me of the joy
you add to my life,
joy that I'm missing… a lot.
So don't forget that I Love you,
that I'm thinking of you,
and that I'm counting every minute
until we're together again.

To my Queen, My Goddess, my External Love Annie
If I were a king,
And you a queen,
And the world our reign,
If I were a God,
And you a Goddess
And the Universe our creation,
How would we feel,
What would we feel,
What would we see,
Only you and me,
If I were time,
And you eternity,
And we spent them together,
How would we love,
With eternal passion,
Only you and me,
I am your lover,
You are my lover,
King and Queen,
God and Goddess,
Time and Eternity,
Together forever,
Only you and me
I Love you my Sweet Little Annie

Text Messages

~ While you Dance with your friends,

~ My heart dances w/ thoughts of how much I Love You

~To Love you more

~ There would have to be 25 hours in the day and 367 days in the year.

~ Every Day remember, how much I Love You....!

~ As Constant as the Stars above Know that You are LOVED!!!!!!!!

~ ILY because of how loved U make me feel.

~ ILY in the morning, ILY each afternoon, ILY @ night because U make me feel so Loved

~ We'll have a competition 2morrow 2 c who loves who more!

~ I just called to say I love you; I just called to say how much I care.

~As Petal to Flower, As Wing to Eagle, As Sunrise to Morning, So You are to ME! Love You Baby - Good Morning

E-mail William sent me while I was in Mexico.

I figured that without a performance tonight you may have some computer time, so here I am. Just a few words that begin and end with how much I Love You. * Maureen is playing a lot of cards; the kids, my daughters, 50 years together, but you hold the most important card, the My Heart and the Love card. I know I have it thoroughly and forever with you. If and when I get a little down, don't get down with me. Hold me in your arms, kiss me, give me the strength to look past the moment and into the future. Two more nights of snuggling with your pillow. Yes, I sleep on my side of the bed, but I find my arms embracing your pillow each morning. It will be wonderful to trade the pillow in for the real thing.

By the way, the Apartment Management was so glad we renewed the lease that they built us our own pool right outside the living room window.

I love you Baby.

William

(Maureen is William's x-wife)

Love Letters and Text Messages to WILLIAM from Annie B

Love Much,
Love in the first light of dawn,
In the last flicker of dusk.
Love every touch, every word,
Each stolen Moment, each playful kiss.
Love every chance to Love and be Loved.
Love long and Love Well.
Just Love~!
I will Love you till......

Do you know what I Love about you?
Do you Know what I Love most about you?
Your Sexy Smile!
No Wait, your cute laugh.
Hold it, your passionate Kisses.
Changed my mind, your warmth and Caring.
I know your sense of Humor.
Even better yet, you're forgiving ways.
Wait, without a doubt, your Gentle touch.
Hold on…..
Now I got it:
You know what I Love most about you?
EVERYTHING
I Love You Baby

To lie Silent
In the Gray of Night,
Watching your slow breaths
Flow in and out,
Rise and Fall,
Your warm skin
Fused with mine
Muscles earlier so tensed
And strained
Now relaxed
In this Twilight World,
This Place of Dreams
Where we Breathe Secrets
No one can Hear.....
" I LOVE YOU"

There is nothing better
In this Life of ours than the first
Consciousness of Love –
The first Fluttering of its silken wings.
Love is an irresistible desire
To be irresistibly desired.
I Love You Baby,

I'm giving you a piece of my heart,
To remind you that I'm always here for you.
No matter how far apart we may be...
I'm giving you a piece of me,
A part of my soul,
That will hold you dearly,
And never let you go...
Whenever you are troubled,
And struggling to smile,
Remember I have a special place for you,
That has no limits and goes on for miles...
There is a part of myself,
That is given to only you,
A place unseen,
That loves you for you...
I'm giving you my Heart
My Sun,
If my heart could talk,
You would know that you've made me strong.
If my heart could move,
It would wrap itself around you,
If my heart could touch,
You would never feel a sweeter Love,
If my heart could talk,
You would understand how deeply,
I LOVE YOU

Loving you is my path.
I never think of the future in terms of where
I'm going – only in terms of where we'll go together.
Loving you is my peace.
It's the quiet satisfaction I feel every time your eyes tell me
That I've listened to you,
Made you happy,
Loved you well.
Loving you is my certainty,
A complete confidence that I'd do anything to give you
The same peace and walk the same path
With you forever.

Weaving together Two Lives
A creation of passion, artistry, and soul.
As long as you live and breathe,
It will continue to evolve into patterns
More intricate and more marvelous
Than either person could render alone.
I miss you and Love you very much

Two become One,
Not by giving up
The Wonderful qualities
That makes them unique individuals,
But by learning, growing,
And becoming whole together.
See you Soon,
I Love You Baby

On the Days
That are summer-sweet
And full of a thousand dreams,
I will Love You
On the Days
When thunder and rain come,
Dashing against our hopes,
I will Love You
On the Days
When we share a quiet world of contentment,
I will Love You
On all the Days
Through all the seasons
Of our Lives,
I will give you my Love,
I will give you my Heart,
I Love You Baby

Love has called our Hearts to Love Flies on Golden Wings
And brings sweet riches
Never dreamed by kings
And oh how beautiful it sings
I Love You Baby
Talk to you in the morning,

This will be an Everlasting Love
Yes this will be an Everlasting Love
This will be the one I've waited for
This will be the first time anyone has Loved me,
I'm so glad you found me in time
And I'm so glad that
That this will be an Everlasting Love
Loving you is Wonderful
Because you've shown me just how much you care
You've give me the thrill of a Lifetime
And made me believe we've got more thrills to come
This will be an Everlasting Love
You've brought a lot of sunshine into my life
You've filled me with happiness I never knew
You gave me more joy than I ever dreamed of
And no one, no one can take the place of you
This will be, yes siree,
Huggin' and squeezin' and kissin'
And pleasin' together forever through rain or whatever
So long as I'm livin' true Love I'll be givin', to you
I Love You Baby

"William You are more than I could ever ask for. I can only hope I am half of what you are someday. You taught me how to care until it hurts, you taught me how to smile again, you even taught me to laugh again. You taught me that life isn't so serious and sometimes you have to play. You have a big, beautiful heart. Through life we need to keep it open and follow it.

"You taught me to never be afraid to be myself. I will always be there in our park. I know someday we will be more together than we are now. You make me smile and shine I hope someday you will really understand what you really did for me. Please don't stop loving life. Take in every breath like it's your first. I will always be there with you. I'll be in the sun, shadows, dreams and joys of your life.

I will always have with me, the feeling of your soft nudges next to me, and the joy I feel when we lay together. "I dream of you every night, and I always will. Don't ever think that when we are not together I didn't love you.

~ Time can change many things, But it will never change my Love for You!

~ Two hearts that share laughter and pain.

Two souls that share Love.

Two minds that help each other grow.

I Love You so Much,
XOXOX till I see you,

~ Home for Love,

A corner for warmth,

A place for Joy.

Love that takes

A Lifetime to Express.

Looking forward to a Lifetime with you

~ Every day we renew

The promises of Love.

In every word or deed

That speaks of Love

Love You

~Dance together

A Dance

No one leads, no one follows,

Each responds to the other.

It is improvised,

The music is always changing…

And it plays forever.

Will you be my forever?

I Love You

~ To give Love

With an open heart,

To honor Love

As the rare gift it is,

To Nurture Love

As you would a tender seedling

Is to know how to make Love Last.

Love You

~ When morning comes,

Love is the Light,

When darkness falls,

Love is the Stars.

I Love you,

~ It is in the Partnership of Love

That we find our Greatest Gifts.

It is in the mirror of Love

That we see our truest selves.

I Love You

~ Only those who Love

Can feel the magic that happens

When two people vow to stay

Lovers forever~!

~ A Small Dwelling

In the wild meadow

Will be enough

If you are there with me.

~ Together is the most beautiful word in the language of Love.

Our Hearts answered Love's soft whisper

~ I just wanted to Wish you a quiet, Comforting Day,

And the Warm feeling that comes from knowing you are Cared about Deeply

Love You

~ I can't wait till I can put my arms around you and give you some Loving.

Just remember that I Love You very Much,

Love Ya,

~ Hello there My Love,

When the sight of that certain face

Or the sound of that special voice

Lightens your heart,

You know your soul is home.

Hope to get to see you soon,

I Love You,

~ How Marvelous it is

To cherish another

Beyond one's self...

And how precious it is

To be so cherished.

Love You,

~ Love is the Caring of Two Hearts,

The pairing of two lives,

The sharing of two souls.

Love you

~ And then big things like Dreams Shared

And problems faced together

Spread the light of Love...

Until the World around

Is bright and beautiful...

Seen through the eyes of Love.

Love You – Double Scoop

~ Love Starts as One Small Flicker in the Heart.

Over time, Kisses, Soft Glances,

And Sweet words fan the Flames.

I Love You

~ Once in a Lifetime,

Right in the middle of an ordinary life,

Love writes a fairy tale.

~ Who knows when it Happens

A smile becomes a sanctuary,

A kiss becomes a taste of heaven,

And a friend becomes a Lover...

Forever

I Love You,

~"One word frees us of all the weight and pain of life: That word is love."

I feel in Love with you again today...

At first there was a simple thought of you

playing over and over in my mind.

Then I smiled...

Remembering the good times,

The tender moments, the love we share,

The relationship we've built together.

All of this made me happy.

And all of those feelings,

That were once so new,

Came rushing back,

And again I fell in Love with you.

We may be miles apart

But I'll be with you wherever you are

I'm already there

Take a look around

I'm the sunshine in your hair

I'm the shadow on the ground

I'm the whisper in the wind

And I'll be there until the end

Can you feel the Love that we share?

Oh I'm already there

I Love You Baby

Love Thoughts by others,

"We love because it's the only true adventure."

"Love is like quicksilver in the hand. Leave the fingers open and it stays. Clutch it, and it darts away."

"Love is friendship set on fire."

"Love is an ideal thing, marriage a real thing."

"To be in love is merely to be in a state of perceptual anesthesia."

"Love is everything it's cracked up to be. That's why people are so cynical about it...It really is worth fighting for, risking everything for. And the trouble is, if you don't risk everything, you risk even more."

"Sometimes love is stronger than a man's convictions."

"Love is the master key that opens the gates of happiness."

"Maybe love is like luck. You have to go all the way to find it."

"Love stretches your heart and makes you big inside."

"Love has no awareness of merit or demerit; it has no scale... Love loves; this is its nature."

"Love is like war: Easy to begin but hard to end."

"Love consists in this, that two solitudes protect and touch and greet each other."

"Where love is, no room is too small."

"Loves makes your soul crawl out from its hiding place."

"Love is the irresistible desire to be irresistibly desired."

"Love is more than three words mumbled before bedtime. Love is sustained by action, a pattern of devotion in the things we do for each other every day."

"To love is to receive a glimpse of heaven."

"A love song is just a caress set to music."

"Love is an act of endless forgiveness, a tender look which becomes a habit."

"Love is like a violin. The music may stop now and then, but the strings remain forever."

"Love is the only sane and satisfactory answer to the problem of human existence."

"In the final analysis, love is the only reflection of man's worth."

"Love doesn't make the world go round, love is what makes the ride worthwhile."

"Oh, life is a glorious cycle of song,
A medley of extemporanea;
And love is a thing that can never go wrong;
And I am Marie of Roumania."

"To love is to suffer. To avoid suffering one must not love. But then one suffers from not loving. Therefore to love is to suffer, not to love is to suffer. To suffer is to suffer. To be happy is to love. To be happy then is to suffer. But suffering makes one unhappy. Therefore, to be unhappy one must love, or love to suffer, or suffer from too much happiness. I hope you're getting this down."

A Daily Reminder for the One I Love

I want you to remember

That true love is forever,

And there is no love truer than

The love I feel for you.

I want you to remember you're

The most wonderful thing

That has happened to me,

My happy ending

My dream come true,

My friend and my love

All wrapped up in one.

I Love You.

How to Get in Touch With Me

If you have other questions or if you are in a similar situation and you would like to talk to somebody just send me an e-mail.

Annieb5747@yahoo.com

I know at times I wished I would have known somebody that I could have just talked with.

So Please feel free to send me an e-mail and we will talk.

Some of my favorite Recipes:

Chicken and Noodle Casserole

1 can Cream of Mushroom Soup
½ cup milk
¼ tsp ground pepper
¼ cup grated Parmesan cheese
1 cup frozen mixed vegetables
2 cups cubed, cooked chicken
½ cup shredded cheddar cheese
2 cups medium egg noodles, cooked and drained

1. Stir everything except the Cheddar Cheese, together, and put in a 1 ½ qt – casserole dish

2. Bake at 400* for 25 minutes or until hot. Stir

3. Top with the Cheddar Cheese

   To make crunchy add 1 cup French Onions

BBQ Bash Party Mix

¼ cup butter melted
2 teaspoons BBQ seasoning, Dry
2 teaspoons liquid smoke
1 teaspoon Worcestershire Sauce
1 teaspoon paprika
1 teaspoon seasoned salt
1/8 teaspoon cayenne pepper
8 cups of your favorite Chex cereal (corn, Rice, and or Wheat)
2 cups BBQ flavored corn chips

1. Preheat oven to 250 F.

2. Combine butter, BBQ seasoning, liquid smoke, Worcestershire Sauce, paprika, seasoned salt and cayenne pepper.

3. Mix well.

4. Gradually add cereal and chips stirring until all pieces are evenly coated.

5. Bake 1 hour stirring every 15 minutes. Once baked spread out on paper towels to cool.

Store in air tight container.

White Chips and Blueberry Bread Pudding

Pudding Mix

1 ¾ cups sugar	1 tablespoon flour
4 eggs	1 stick (1/2 cup) unsalted butter softened
1 cup buttermilk	1 tablespoon lime juice
2 tablespoons vanilla	1 bag of White Chocolate chips

1 ½ cups frozen Blueberries
½ loaf of white bread cut into cubes (enough to fill a 13x9 pan)

1. Preheat oven to 350 F butter a 13x9 glass baking dish.

2. Beat eggs slightly add the flour and sugar, blending well. Mix in the butter, then add the buttermilk and blend with whisk. Add lime juice and vanilla. Blend well. Add the chips and blueberries. Spread the bread in the baking dish and pour the filling over the bread, mix a little to get the filling on all the bread. Let the mixture set for 10 minutes, so the bread will absorb all the liquid.

3. Bake for about 30 minutes or until the top is brown.

Amaretto topping

1 tablespoon cornstarch   *¼ cup Amaretto Liqueur*
1 ½ cups heavy cream   *¾ cup sugar*

1. In small bowl dissolve the cornstarch in the liqueur and whisk until smooth.

2. In medium saucepan, scald cream over medium heat.

3. Add the liqueur mixture to the hot cream and whisking constantly, bring to a boil.

4. Reduce heat and cook, whisking for 30 second. Remove from heat and add the sugar. Whisk until dissolved. Let cool to room temperature before serving over bread pudding.

First Class Coconut Cake

Cake
1 yellow cake mix
1 small box vanilla instant pudding
1 1/3 cups water
4 eggs
¼ cup oil
2 cups coconut
1 cup pecans

1. Mix everything expect coconut and pecans together until smooth, then add coconut and pecans. Bake at 350 F for 35 minutes.

Frosting
2 cups coconut
2 tablespoons butter – softened
1 – 8 oz cream cheese – softened
2 teaspoons milk
1 box powder sugar
½ teaspoon vanilla

1. Mix everything except coconut until smooth. Mix in coconut.

Texas Cow Chip Cookies

2 cups butter (room
temperature)

2 cups white sugar

2 cups brown sugar

4 eggs

2 tablespoons vanilla

4 cups flour

½ teaspoon salt

2 teaspoons baking powder

2 teaspoons baking soda

2 cups oatmeal

2 cups corn flakes

2 cups chopped pecans

2 cups flaked coconut

2 cups raisins

2 – 12 oz. pkgs Chocolate
Chips

1 – 12 oz pkg peanut butter
chips

1. In a VERY LARGE MIXING BOWL – beat butter
   and sugars together. Until well blended. Add eggs
   and beat until smooth. Stir in vanilla.

2. In a separate bowl, combine flour, salt, baking soda
   and baking powder. Gradually add to the sugar
   mixture and stir well. Stir in remaining ingredients
   in order.

3. Drop cookies with a ¼ measuring cup onto lightly
   greased cookie sheet. For best results don't over
   crowd the cookies, leave lots of room between them,
   they will grow.

4. Bake at 350 F for 12-15 minutes.

Volcano Cake

German chocolate cake mix
1 c chopped pecans
1 cup flaked coconut
10 Almond Joy candy Bars
1 8oz package cream cheese
1 stick unsalted butter
1 c powdered sugar

1. Grease and flour a 9 x 13 pan

2. Cover bottom of pan with pecans and coconut.

3. Make German chocolate cake mix according to package.

4. Cut up candy bars into bite sized pieces and add to the batter, pour over the coconut pecan mixture.

5. Mix together cream cheese, butter, and powdered sugar.

6. Dollop over the cake mix.

7. Bake at 350 F for 50 minutes, Yummy!

Pumpkin Cheesecake

2 – 8 oz pkgs of Cream Cheese – softened
½ cup sugar
½ cup canned pumpkin
½ teaspoon vanilla
½ teaspoon ground cinnamon
Dash each – ground cloves and nutmeg
2 eggs
1 Graham Cracker Crust

1. Mix cream cheese, pumpkin, sugar, vanilla, and spices at medium speed with electric mixer until smooth.

2. Add eggs, mix until smooth.

3. Pour into crust – sprinkle remaining chips on top

4. Bake at 350 F for 40 minutes or until center is almost set. Cool. Refrigerate overnight.

5. Top with whip cream.

Peppermint Stick Cheesecake

2 – 8 oz pkgs of Cream Cheese – softened
½ cup sugar
½ teaspoon vanilla
2 eggs
1 cup finely crushed peppermint candy
1 Graham Cracker Crust

1. Mix cream cheese, sugar, and vanilla at medium speed with electric mixer until smooth.

2. Add eggs, mix until smooth. Stir in ¾ cup of peppermint.

3. Pour into crust – sprinkle remaining candy on top

4. Bake at 350 F for 40 minutes or until center is almost set. Cool. Refrigerate overnight.

Chocolate Chip Cheesecake

2 – 8 oz pkgs of Cream Cheese – softened
½ cup sugar
½ teaspoon vanilla
2 eggs
1 pkg of Chocolate Chips
1 Graham Cracker Crust

1. Mix cream cheese, sugar, and vanilla at medium speed with electric mixer until smooth.

2. Add eggs, mix until smooth. Stir in ¾ bag of chips.

3. Pour into crust – sprinkle remaining chips on top

4. Bake at 350 F for 40 minutes or until center is almost set. Cool. Refrigerate overnight.

Pralines and Cream Cheesecake

2 – 8 oz pkgs of Cream Cheese – softened
½ cup sugar
½ teaspoon vanilla
2 eggs
1 cup almond brickle chips
1 Graham Cracker Crust
3 tablespoons caramel ice cream topping

1. Mix cream cheese, sugar, and vanilla at medium speed with electric mixer until smooth.

2. Add eggs, mix until smooth. Stir in almond brickle chips.

3. Pour into crust – pour caramel topping over the top then run knife slowly over top just to lightly give it a marble look.

4. Bake at 350 F for 40 minutes or until center is almost set. Cool. Refrigerate overnight.

Onion Dip

2 pkg cream cheese
1 cup mayo
1 cup grated parmesan cheese
1 large white onion chopped – (nickel size)

1. Mix all together. Bake at 350 F about 35 minutes.
2. Serve with chips or crackers

Texas Two-Step Slaw

6 cups shredded green cabbage
2 cups shredded red cabbage
1 cup chopped green onion
2 pickled jalapenos finely chopped
2 tablespoons chopped cilantro
1 can fiesta corn drained
1 cup shredded cheddar cheese

Combine all in large bowl

Dressing:
¾ cup Ranch Dressing
1 tablespoon lime juice
1 teaspoon ground cumin
1 tablespoon sugar

Mix the dressing and add to the salad mix, right before serving

Sweet Potato Casserole

3 cups Sweet Potatoes
½ cup sugar
1 teaspoon vanilla
1 teaspoon allspice
½ cup butter
1/3 cup milk
1 teaspoon cinnamon
2 eggs
1 ½ teaspoon nutmeg

Boil, drain, and mash potatoes, mix in sugar, spices, butter, eggs, vanilla, and milk. Put in 13x9 baking dish.

Topping:
1/3 melted butter
1 cup chopped pecans
1 cup light brown sugar
½ cup flour

1. Melt butter and mix remaining ingredients, sprinkle on top of potato mixture.

2. Bake 25 minutes at 350 F

Western Baked Beans

¾ cup brown sugar
3 cans pork-n-beans
½ cup vinegar
Salt and pepper
½ teaspoon mustard
Dash Worcestershire sauce
1 can lima beans
¾ cup molasses
1 can butter beans
1 chopped onion
1 can kidney beans
1 pound fried bacon – crumbled
1 pound ground beef – browned
1 large can tomatoes

Simmer the brown sugar, vinegar, and mustard in large pot. Once all mixed add everything else. Cook on top of stove on medium heat for about 1 hour.

<u>Corn Casserole</u>

2 cans Mexicorn – drained
1 pound Velveeta Cheese
1 ½ cup uncooked rice – cooked
1 can cream of mushroom soup

1. Cook rice and mix all together, bake at 350 F for about 25 minutes.
2. Look for the cheese to be melted.

Lickety Split Spoons

1 cup semi-sweet Chocolate chips   1 cup white chocolate chips
   1 cup mint chocolate chips   72 colored plastic spoons
       Candy Decorations:
    Crushed hard peppermint   Colored Sugar crystals

1. Melt chocolate's in heavy 1 quart sauce pans, over the lowest possible heat stirring – constantly

2. Dip spoons into melted chocolate coating only the bowl of the spoon. Sprinkle with candy decorations while the chocolate is still wet. Place spoons on waxed paper until chocolate is firm.

Pumpkin Pie

¾ cup sugar
½ teaspoon salt
1 ¾ teaspoon Pumpkin Pie Spice
2 large eggs
1 can 100% Pure Pumpkin
1 can Carnation Evaporated Milk
1 unbaked Pie Shell

1. Mix sugar, salt, and pumpkin pie spice in small bowl. Beat eggs in large bowl, stir in pumpkin and sugar, spice mixture. Gradually stir in Evaporated milk. Pour into pie shell.

2. Bake 425 F for 15 minutes – then reduce heat to 350 F and bake for 40 minutes or until knife inserted comes out clean.

3. Cool for 2 hours

Yummy Chocolate Cake

Melt in Double Boiler:
½ cup Wesson oil
1 cup water
½ cup butter

Combine the following:

2 cups all purpose flour	2 cups sugar
4 tablespoons cocoa	1 teaspoon baking powder
2 eggs	½ cup buttermilk
1 teaspoon vanilla	

DO NOT Use Mixer with this cake.

1. Butter and flour pan (13x9)
2. Bake for 25 – 30 minutes

Icing

Melt in double boiler

1 stick butter	4 tablespoons cocoa
3 tablespoons milk	¾ box powdered sugar

Ice Cake while Icing is HOT

Holiday Peppermint Bark

1 pkg white chocolate chips
1 cup peppermint – crushed

1. Line the counter with Wax paper – microwave white chocolate in microwave safe bowl for just a few seconds at a time until all is melted and smooth – not to long at one time or it will burn the chocolate.

2. Add crushed peppermint and stir. Pour candy out on wax paper – spread to about the thickness of 2 coins together.

3. Let it set and get firm for about an hour, then break it up into bite size pieces, store in air tight container at room temperature.

Taco Stew

1 ½ pound ground beef – browned
1 large onion –chopped
1 Bell Pepper – chopped
2 cans tomatoes – chopped
1 can Rotel tomatoes
2 pkg Dry Hidden Valley Ranch Mix
1 pkg Dry Taco Seasoning Mix
1 can Ranch Style Beans
1 garlic clove - chopped
1 can corn

1. In large pot add browned beef, onions, and peppers mix well.
2. Add everything else except corn, (wait till the stew is almost ready before you add the corn)
3. Rinse each can out with a little water (1/2 can) and add to stew.
4. Bring to a boil, cover and let it set – then add corn.

Chilies Relleno's Casserole

1 can 7 oz – whole green chilies
1 ½ cup 6 oz – shredded Colby / Monterey Jack Cheese
¾ pound ground beef
¼ cup chopped onion
1 cup milk
4 eggs
¼ cup all-purpose flour
¼ teaspoon salt
¼ teaspoon pepper
Brown beef with onion.

1. Split chilies and remove seeds; dry on paper towel.

2. Arrange chilies on bottom of greased 2 quart dish top with cheese, spoon the browned beef and onion over the cheese.

3. In mixing bowl, beat milk, eggs, flour, salt and pepper until smooth;

4. Pour over chilies and beef mixture.

5. Bake uncovered at 350 F 40 – 45 minutes or until knife comes out clean.

<u>Sweet – n – Sour Meatballs</u>

<u>Meatballs:</u>
1 pound ground beef
½ cup Dry Bread crumbs
¼ cup milk
3 tablespoons finely chopped onion
1 teaspoon salt
1 teaspoon Worcestershire Sauce
1 egg

Mix all together make small balls, place on cookies sheet and bake at 400 F until light brown.

<u>Sauce:</u>
½ cup packed brown sugar
1 tablespoon cornstarch
1 can 13 oz – pineapple chunks
1/3 cup vinegar
1 tablespoon soy sauce
Small green pepper – chopped

1. Mix brown sugar and cornstarch in pan, stir in pineapples with juice, vinegar, and soy sauce. Heat to boiling, stirring, reduce heat add meatballs.
2. Simmer 10 minutes – serve over Rice

Pork Chop Casserole

4-5 pork chops
6 beef bouillon cubes
3 cups HOT water
5 potatoes - cubed
Salt and Pepper

1. Lightly brown pork chops in skillet with salt and pepper.
2. Place pork chops and potatoes in baking pan pour hot water in pan then drop in bouillon cubes. Bake at 350 F for 45 minutes.

Chicken Taco's

Whole chicken – cooked – shredded
½ cup Picante sauce
½ cup onion – chopped
½ teaspoon ground cumin
1 cup cheddar cheese – shredded
Lettuce, Tomatoes

Combine everything, warm and serve in taco shells

Chicken Spaghetti

1 whole chicken – cooked – shredded
Small pkg spaghetti – cooked – drained
1 small onion – chopped
1 can cream of mushroom
1 can cream of celery
1 can cheddar cheese soup
2 cups cheddar cheese – shredded

1. Mix everything together except shredded cheese – pour in baking dish.

2. Top with shredded cheese.

3. Bake until cheese is all melted.

Chicken Tortilla Bake

3 cups chicken – cooked – shredded
2 cans – 4 oz- chopped green chilies
1 cup chicken broth
1 can cream of mushroom soup
1 can cream of chicken soup
1 small onion – finely chopped
12 corn tortillas
2 cups shredded – cheddar cheese

1. In bowl combine the chicken, chilies, broth, soups and onion; set aside.

2. Warm tortillas, layer ½ of them in bottom of a greased baking pan, top w ½ of the chicken mixture, ½ of the cheese, then repeat.

3. Bake uncovered at 350F for 30 minutes.

Acorn Squash Casserole

Acorn squashes - as many as you need for the number of people you are serving. Keep in mind that the amount of usable squash that you scrape out of the husk is considerably less than the size of the vegetable.

1. Cut the squash in half. Sprinkle with Maple Syrup.

2. Bake until fork goes into meat of squash easily. About 25-40 minutes depending on the size of the acorn squash.

3. 1 Large onion diced and sautéed in one stick of butter until starting to brown lightly. Scoop the squash out of the shell. Mash with a potato masher. Add onions with remaining butter.

4. Mix and enjoy.

I sprinkled lightly with brown sugar/ cinnamon during the mixing for extra flavor.

www.ingramcontent.com/pod-product-compliance
Lightning Source LLC
Chambersburg PA
CBHW061349280526
45784CB00001B/193